Register Now for Online Access to Your Book!

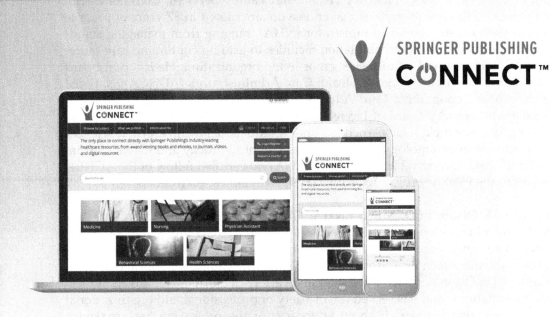

SPRINGER PUBLISHING
CONNECT™

Your print purchase of *The Health Services Executive (HSE™) Q&A Review*
includes online access to the contents of your book—increasing accessibility,
portability, and searchability!

Access today at:
http://connect.springerpub.com/content/book/978-0-8261-3526-1
or scan the QR code at the right with your smartphone
and enter the access code below.

L7BE1JY0

*Scan here for
quick access.*

**If you are experiencing problems accessing the digital component of this product,
please contact our customer service department at cs@springerpub.com**

The online access with your print purchase is available at the publisher's discretion and may be
removed at any time without notice.

Publisher's Note: New and used products purchased from third-party sellers are not guaranteed for
quality, authenticity, or access to any included digital components.

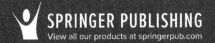

SPRINGER PUBLISHING
View all our products at springerpub.com

Keith R. Knapp, PhD, MHA, HSE, CFACHCA, currently serves as associate professor in the Department of Health Management and Policy at the University of Kentucky's College of Public Health and as senior adviser on Adult Programs to the secretary of the Cabinet for Health and Family Services, Commonwealth of Kentucky. His current professional endeavors are rooted in 37 years of practice as a licensed nursing home administrator (NHA), ranging from managing stand-alone skilled nursing and rehabilitation facilities to leading continuing care retirement communities and a multi-site senior living organization. He is a past board chair of the American College of Health Care Administrators (ACHCA); National Association of Long Term Care Administrator Boards (NAB) and its affiliated foundation, Kentucky Board of Licensure for Long-Term Care Administrators; and LeadingAge (Kentucky). He earned his undergraduate degree in arts and sciences and doctorate in gerontology from the University of Kentucky and his MHA from Xavier (Ohio) University. He is a licensed NHA and certified fellow of the ACHCA and holds the Health Services Executive (HSE™) qualification from the NAB.

Douglas M. Olson, PhD, MBA, LNHA, FACHCA, is director of the Center for Health Administration and Aging Services Excellence (CHAASE) and professor of health administration at the University of Wisconsin–Eau Claire (UWEC). Prior to his academic career, Dr. Olson devoted 12 years to leading long-term care communities. Dr. Olson has been published in a variety of journals, has given numerous presentations, and has served on a variety of professional and organizational boards. His current research about advocacy for the profession has sparked a national collaboration among senior living organizations, academic programs, trade and professional associations, consumers, and regulatory agencies to mount a coordinated effort to properly prepare enough future leaders in this field to meet the anticipated demand—known as Vision 2025. He earned his BS in healthcare administration from UWEC, MBA from the University of St. Thomas, and PhD in health services administration, research, and policy from the University of Minnesota. He is a licensed nursing home administrator (NHA) and fellow of the American College of Health Care Administrators (ACHCA).

The Health Services Executive (HSE™) Q&A Review

Keith R. Knapp, PhD, MHA, HSE, CFACHCA

Douglas M. Olson, PhD, MBA, LNHA, FACHCA

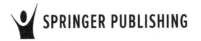

Springer Publishing Company, LLC
11 West 42nd Street, New York, NY 10036
www.springerpub.com
connect.springerpub.com/

Acquisitions Editor: David D'Addona
Compositor: Amnet Systems

ISBN: 978-0-8261-3525-4
ebook ISBN: 978-0-8261-3526-1
DOI: 10.1891/9780826135261

21 22 23 24 25 / 5 4 3 2 1

The author and the publisher of this Work have made every effort to use sources believed to be reliable to provide information that is accurate and compatible with the standards generally accepted at the time of publication. The author and publisher shall not be liable for any special, consequential, or exemplary damages resulting, in whole or in part, from the readers' use of, or reliance on, the information contained in this book. The publisher has no responsibility for the persistence or accuracy of URLs for external or third-party Internet websites referred to in this publication and does not guarantee that any content on such websites is, or will remain, accurate or appropriate.

Library of Congress Cataloging-in-Publication Data

Names: Knapp, Keith R., author. | Olson, Douglas M., author.
Title: The health services executive (HSE) Q&A review / Keith R. Knapp, Douglas M. Olson.
Other titles: Health services executive (HSE) Q & A review
Description: New York, NY : Springer Publishing Company, LLC, [2021] | Includes bibliographical references and index.
Identifiers: LCCN 2020050125 (print) | LCCN 2020050126 (ebook) | ISBN 9780826135254 (paperback) | ISBN 9780826135261 (ebook)
Subjects: MESH: Health Facility Administrators | Health Services Administration | Leadership | United States | Examination Questions
Classification: LCC RA971 (print) | LCC RA971 (ebook) | NLM WX 18.2 | DDC 362.1068—dc23
LC record available at https://lccn.loc.gov/2020050125
LC ebook record available at https://lccn.loc.gov/2020050126

Contact us to receive discount rates on bulk purchases.
We can also customize our books to meet your needs.
For more information please contact: sales@springerpub.com

Publisher's Note: New and used products purchased from third-party sellers are not guaranteed for quality, authenticity, or access to any included digital components.

Printed in the United States of America.

I dedicate my contributions to this text to my lovely wife, Jane, without whose love, support, encouragement, and patience throughout the writing and editing process I would have faltered; to my family—parents, siblings, children, and grandchildren—who inspired my drive to share valuable lived experiences with the next generations; and to the nation's senior living organizations, their consumers, staff members, and families of both.

—K2

I dedicate my contributions to this text to my son, Lukas, who tolerated evenings when his dad was on his computer rather than playing another game of one-on-one hoops in the driveway; to my mom, whose quiet selfless devotion to her family and long-term care nursing career taught me how to balance the best of both; to my immediate and extended family, who always valued the wisdom of elders and the joy of young ones; and to the colleagues I have been blessed to get to know and be inspired by over the years.

—DO

Contents

Acknowledgments

Several widely recognized leaders in the field of senior living leadership have offered insightful comments, recommendations, observations, and opinions concerning a host of topics, which have helped us shape this resource. David D'Addona and Jaclyn Shultz have been extraordinarily helpful in shepherding this project, as have been the editorial and production staff at Springer Publishing Company. Our colleagues at the University of Kentucky and University of Wisconsin–Eau Claire (UWEC) have consistently provided encouragement and scheduling flexibility throughout the process, affording us the professional space and time to complete it. The UWEC healthcare administration students devoted some of their time to gathering related resources and exploring concepts that helped inform the development of the textbook and this companion Q&A resource. Our peers in academe, who teach courses regarding senior living leadership and long-term care administration, have clamored for new texts, which truly reflect the current environment, and have supported our attempt at producing one that is relevant and rooted in practice. We are extremely grateful to all!

CHAPTER 1

Introduction to the HSE™ Exam

The field of senior care is changing in a variety of ways because of demographic shifts, consumer preferences, available resources, government policies, and other factors. The changing landscape will likely continue to evolve over time. The responsibility of the profession is to stay as current as possible with the preparation of leaders to navigate this continuum of care and services in a variety of places and settings. Educators must attempt to offer content and material that is as close to the current realities and projected futures of the field as possible.

One of the ways that this is accomplished is by practice analyses conducted by agencies and associations in the field. In the senior care space, the National Association of Long Term Care Administrator Boards (NAB) conducts a professional practice analysis about every 5 to 7 years to determine the knowledge and skills a person should possess to lead a senior care organization, referred to as its *domains of practice*. All states license nursing home administrators. Many are beginning to also license or consider licensing administrators of residential care/assisted living (RC/AL) facilities and some home- and community-based (HCBS) lines of service. The NAB recently commissioned a study that suggested that four out of five of the skills and knowledge areas included in its established domains were comparable across multiple lines of service. That served as the basis for the NAB's development of the Health Services Executive (HSE™) qualification, which is a credential that allows individuals to practice along the continuum of health services and supports and enhances the portability of their administrator license. This is not in place of a state-issued professional license, but it is an advanced credential enabling licensure boards to offer licensure by equivalency to those who have earned it. The NAB offers career and education pathways to meet the qualifications needed to apply for the HSE™, both of which require examinations to assess competency (NAB, 2020). At the time of this initial publication, nearly half of the NAB member licensure boards across the country have adopted the HSE™ credential for granting licensure by equivalency.

The evolving field of senior care services has a variety of other organizations involved in leadership development. Two examples of the expanding areas of the profession include AL communities and home care agencies. The work of the Senior Living Certification Commission that developed a Director of Assisted Living certification program sponsored by Argentum has also been considered in the formation of this resource. Additionally, the National Association for Home Care & Hospice has an independent, advanced certification program for individuals in leadership positions that leads to designation as a Certified Home Care and Hospice Executive. These efforts and others will continue and should be paid attention to as the market and profession continue to shift to meet the changing demand and preferences of seniors and adults with disabilities and the corresponding preparation needs for leaders of organizations serving them.

The Health Services Executive (HSE™) Q&A Review provides a comprehensive and practical study tool for all students and professionals seeking HSE™ qualification. This resource helps an individual assess their knowledge and competency in a variety of established areas and across the postacute continuum of care and services. Divided into two parts, this resource allows readers to test their knowledge in each area covered by the HSE™ exam established by the NAB.

Part I features multiple-choice, single-best-answer questions grouped by domain of practice—customer care, supports, and services; human resources; finance; environment; and management and leadership—with rationales accompanying each "best" answer. Part II simulates the exam, offering a separate exam for the Core of Knowledge content and each of the three lines of service: nursing home administration (NHA), RC/AL, and HCBS. These exams are structured to model the current content blueprint of the NAB licensure exams. Part III provides the best-answer rationales to enhance self-assessment and further learning in corresponding chapters. The NAB's 2020 practice analysis is approaching completion at the time of this work's publication. Based on the outcomes of previous practice analyses, subtle shifts are expected in the weights assigned to each domain and/or domain characteristics.

Drawing upon the most current information available and written by leading experts in the senior care and services administration field, this Q&A review is one of the most authoritative and comprehensive available. This resource contains over 470 questions with best-answer rationales. It is a must-have supplemental resource for leaders in the field, whether they are taking their initial licensure exams or completing the remaining lines of service exams. The goal of helping and supporting future leaders to understand their competency more fully is a fundamental foundation for their development and success as future leaders of organizations entrusted to provide care and service for the deserving seniors and adults with disabilities in our country.

For more information on how to qualify for the exam or to see frequently asked questions, please visit the following websites:

www.nabweb.org/health-services-executive
www.nabweb.org/filebin/pdf/HSE_FAQ.pdf

RESOURCES

Argentum. (2020). *Certified Director of Assisted Living.* https://www.argentum.org/assisted-living-executive-director-certification-program/

National Association for Home Care & Hospice. (2020). *Certified Home Care and Hospice Executive.* https://www.nahc.org/chce/

National Association of Long Term Care Administrator Boards. (2020). *Health Services Executive.* https://www.nabweb.org/health-services-executive

Practice Questions

CHAPTER 2

Customer Care, Supports, and Services (NAB Domain 1)

1. More Americans aged 65 and over die from _____ than any other cause.
   A. Stroke
   B. Chronic obstructive pulmonary disease (COPD)
   C. Diabetes
   D. Heart disease

2. The foundational therapy disciplines in the postacute care continuum are considered to be physical therapy (PT), speech-language pathology and audiology, and _____.
   A. Occupational therapy
   B. Pet therapy
   C. Music and art therapies
   D. Aquatic therapy

3. The subspecialty of physical therapy (PT) with a focus on the unique movement needs and capabilities of older adults is known as _____ PT.
   A. Gerontological
   B. Geriatric
   C. Restorative
   D. Eldercare

4. A physical therapy (PT) assistant works under the direct supervision of a licensed physical therapist, and a physical therapist aide can work under the direct supervision of either a licensed physical therapist or a _____.
   A. PT practitioner
   B. Physician assistant
   C. PT assistant
   D. Chiropractor

5. The compliance component of the CMS's (Centers for Medicare & Medicaid Services') "Five-Star Quality Rating System" for skilled nursing facilities encompasses the _____ most recent Medicare/Medicaid certification inspections.
   A. Three
   B. Two
   C. Four
   D. Five

6. The compliance component of the Centers for Medicare & Medicaid Services' (CMS's) "Five-Star Quality Rating System" for skilled nursing facilities places the greatest weight on _____.
   A. The Life Safety Code compliance report
   B. The most recent Medicare/Medicaid inspections
   C. The inspections with the greatest number of cited deficiencies
   D. The scope and severity of the last state licensure survey

7. The clinical interdisciplinary team (IDT) blends the expertise of people with complementary professional backgrounds, knowledge, and skills to accomplish each of the following except _____.
   A. Thoroughly assessing a person's condition
   B. Determining the facility's Medicaid rate
   C. Identifying problems or needs
   D. Developing a comprehensive plan of care

8. The interdisciplinary team's core membership for a skilled nursing facility, inpatient rehabilitation facility, and home health agency services typically includes a physician (or licensed designee), a nurse, a social worker, therapists (physical therapy/occupational therapy/speech therapy), and _____.
   A. A medical records coordinator
   B. A housekeeper
   C. A pharmacist
   D. A dietitian

9. Coordination of the interdisciplinary team (IDT) is paramount—scheduling, information sharing, assigning and monitoring workflow, and documenting progress—for establishing and achieving clinical care goals and for _____.
   A. Mission advancement
   B. Optimizing reimbursement
   C. Regulatory compliance
   D. Minimizing rework

10. Accurate and timely documentation is required to ensure quality of care, evaluate opportunities for performance improvement, and validate _____.
    A. Reimbursement rates
    B. Care plan goals
    C. Census
    D. Assessment skills

11. Because the average length of stay in a hospital currently _____, a customer's exposure to the organization is generally limited to the most visible services, such as medical and nursing care, therapies, dining services, chaplaincy, and social services.
    A. Extends for a few weeks
    B. Falls short of 1 week
    C. Varies greatly
    D. Lasts just over 9 days

12. Senior consumers typically want to receive care from personnel who are respectful, friendly, available, and _____.
    A. Energetic
    B. Loud enough
    C. Competent
    D. Polite

13. Senior living is moving from a medical, institution-centric model of service toward a more person-centered, social model of service, with increasing emphasis on _____.
    A. The value proposition
    B. Quality of life over quantity of life
    C. Balancing compliance with autonomy
    D. Recipient-defined expectations

14. _____ protects the public's interest by establishing professional standards of practice on which people can rely in selecting a service provider.
    A. Credentialing
    B. The U.S. Department of Education
    C. The Office of Inspector General
    D. Medicare.gov

15. In healthcare and senior living, professional competence generally refers to _____ established _____ standards of knowledge and skills to practice in a specific discipline.
    A. Upholding, advanced
    B. Exceeding, examination
    C. Embracing, quality
    D. Meeting, minimum

16. A person who already holds an academic degree and wants to learn more about a particular subject, such as gerontology or accounting, but do so without acquiring another degree might earn a _____ from an academic program that offers such an option.
    A. Diploma
    B. Certificate
    C. Plaque
    D. Recognition

17. _____ is typically awarded by a nongovernmental organization, generally a professional membership society that represents the interests of that profession, to someone who demonstrates advanced proficiency in their discipline.
    A. Certification
    B. Licensure
    C. Fellowship
    D. Accreditation

18. The underlying premise of self-directed work teams is that _____.
    A. Small group problem-solving increases efficiency
    B. It is the most effective union prevention method
    C. The people most affected by a decision will be better at making it
    D. Performance improvement offsets the staff time invested

19. Virginia Bell and David Troxel, creators of the "Best Friends™ Approach to Dementia Care," coined the term "the Knack" as a central element in their formula for success in serving persons with Alzheimer's disease and related disorders, which includes an attitude and a set of skills that entail knowledge, nurturing, approach, community, and _____.
    A. Kinship
    B. Stamina
    C. Compassion
    D. Flexibility

20. The health services executive should understand, proactively plan, and effectively execute _____.
    A. Articles of incorporation
    B. Corporate bylaws
    C. Bond covenants
    D. Person-centered change

21. The concept of total quality management (TQM) encompasses at least eight core principles, all of which can effectively be applied to the senior living field: (a) customer-centered service, (b) employee engagement, (c) ongoing process improvement, (d) quality assurance and performance improvement, (e) interdisciplinary coordination and collaboration, (f) strategic and systematic approach, (g) effective communication, and (h) _____.
    A. Consistently fair and equal treatment
    B. Evidence-based decision-making
    C. Advocacy for customers and their families
    D. Commitment to competitive compensation

22. Which of the following is *not* an example of a clinical outcome measure that could serve as a critical success factor in determining quality of care in a senior living setting?
    A. Medication errors
    B. Preventable rehospitalizations
    C. Average length of stay
    D. Infection rates

23. Hospital Corporation of America (HCA) developed an iterative performance improvement process that sets the stage for employing the Deming (Plan–Do–Check–Act) cycle: (a) find a process to improve, (b) organize the effort to work on the improvement, (c) clarify knowledge of the process, (d) understand process variation, and (e) _____.
    A. Start the PDSA (Plan–Do–Study–Act) cycle
    B. Stop identified rework
    C. Select a strategy for improvement
    D. Sample the revised process or outcome

24. The _____ process is a simple problem-solving technique that can prove useful in conducting a root cause analysis by repeatedly questioning what caused the issue.
    A. Five whys
    B. Fishbone diagram
    C. Capillary connectivity
    D. Derivative digging

25. The National Association of Long Term Care Administrator Boards (NAB) calls the domain that involves knowledge and skills about planning, developing, implementing, monitoring, and evaluating all services based on care recipient preferences and assessed needs, as well as compliance with applicable federal and state rules and regulations, _____.
    A. Clinical services management
    B. Resident and client care
    C. Culture change leadership
    D. Customer care, supports, and services

26. Common elements of root cause analyses include the development of an array of possible contributors to and influences on the identified problem, a focus on a particular process point for intervention, the selection of a solution, _____, and a measurement process for determining whether the action works or needs further refinement.
    A. A cost–benefit analysis
    B. A proceed-or-halt decision
    C. A cost estimate
    D. Implementation

27. The two leading professional associations to which a senior living organization's director of nursing or health services should consider belonging are The National Association of Directors of Nursing Administration in Long-Term Care (NADONA/LTC) and the _____.
    A. American Association of Directors of Nursing Services (AADNS)
    B. National Society for Gerontological Nursing
    C. Geriatrics Society of America
    D. Aging Life Care Association

28. A progressive health services executive will encourage and support nursing assistants or nurse aides joining and actively participating in the _____.
   A. American Nurses Association
   B. American Health Care Association
   C. National Association of Health Care Assistants (NAHCA)
   D. LeadingAge

29. The nation's largest association of postacute care providers, which advocates for quality care and services for frail, elderly, and disabled Americans by representing the long-term care community to government, business leaders, and the public, is _____.
   A. LeadingAge
   B. The American Health Care Association (AHCA)
   C. Argentum
   D. Senior Care Providers United

30. Originally established by like-minded, not-for-profit, and faith-based providers of long-term care and senior housing from around the nation as the American Association of Homes for the Aging, it is now known as _____.
   A. LeadingAge
   B. The American Health Care Association
   C. Argentum
   D. The National Council on the Aging

ANSWERS AND RATIONALES

1. Answer: **D.** According to the Centers for Disease Control and Prevention, the leading causes of death among Americans aged 65 and over are (in descending order) as follows: heart disease, cancer, COPD, stroke, Alzheimer's disease, diabetes, pneumonia and flu, and accidents.

2. Answer: **A.** Pet, music, art, and aquatic therapies are considered emerging therapy disciplines in senior living; foundational or core therapies are more commonly recognized by third-party payers as critical for treatment and included in reimbursement models.

3. Answer: **B.** "Geriatric PT" is the term applied by the American Physical Therapy Association for this subspecialty.

4. Answer: **C.** A PT assistant completes more formal training and has broader caregiving duties than a PT aide, often including supervision of one or more PT aides.

5. Answer: **A.** The CMS is interested in both a performance snapshot and monitoring performance trends.

6. Answer: **B.** The CMS expects performance improvement from providers, so greater weight is assigned to more recent evaluations.

7. Answer: **B.** Although the IDT's effort may help establish the aggregate resident acuity—or case mix—its primary responsibility is not financial reimbursement.

8. Answer: **D.** Nutrition is a key factor in both wellness and life satisfaction.

9. Answer: **C.** All members of the IDT must understand what is expected, perform their respective assignments, and hold one another accountable—for the benefit of the resident and in order to meet or exceed regulatory requirements.

10. Answer: **A.** Reimbursement must appropriately reflect the level of services provided, which in turn must match each care recipient's needs—the written record serves as an attestation that the services were needed and delivered.

11. Answer: **B.** According to the Organisation for Economic Coordination and Development, the average length of stay in an American hospital in 2017 was 5.5 days.

12. Answer: **C.** Consumer confidence starts with how well the caregiver can perform the duties of the job—do they know what to do and how?

13. Answer: **D.** Understanding what the consumer wants—not just what they may need—is paramount in delivering truly person-centered care and services.

14. Answer: **A.** Objective, third-party validation of one's knowledge and skills to perform the services of a health profession is critical to public protection.

15. Answer: **D.** Healthcare regulations and standards typically set a minimum level for performance that is acceptable.

16. Answer: **B.** Certificate programs typically include highly focused content about a discipline or subspecialty within a discipline.

17. Answer: **A.** Certification validates a health professional's mastery of advanced proficiency in a particular skill.

18. Answer: **C.** People who are closest to the care recipient—to the work and services—typically have the most relevant knowledge about the opportunities for improvement.

19. Answer: **A.** Kinship represents a family-like tie and genuine concern.

20. Answer: **D.** Person-centered change requires intentional action by the organization's leader; the alternate response options call for corporate compliance, but not necessarily with the goal of change.

21. Answer: **B.** Evidence-based decision-making is more essential to TQM than any of the alternate response options.

22. Answer: **C.** Each of the alternate response options is a clinical outcome measure.

23. Answer: **C.** HCA's performance improvement model is known as FOCUS-PDSA. Selecting a strategy for the improvement is the "S."

24. Answer: **A.** Five whys (or 5 whys) is an iterative interrogative technique used to explore the cause-and-effect relationships underlying a particular problem. The primary goal of the technique is to determine the root cause of a defect or problem by repeating the question "Why?"

25. Answer: **D.** According to the NAB Candidate Handbook, available at www .nabweb.org/filebin/pdf/NAB_Handbook_October_2019_WEB.pdf.

26. Answer: **D.** Implementation is a key element of root cause analysis.

27. Answer: **A.** Both NADONA/LTC and AADNS represent the interests of senior living clinical leadership personnel.

28. Answer: **C.** The mission of the NAHCA is to elevate the professional standing and performance of caregivers through recognition, advocacy, education, and empowerment while building a strong alliance with healthcare providers to maximize success and quality patient care; investing in membership sends a message of keen interest in staff development at every level.

29. Answer: **B.** AHCA members provide essential care to approximately 1 million individuals in over 14,000 facilities.

30. Answer: **A.** The association changed its name in 2010 to LeadingAge.

CHAPTER 3

Human Resources (NAB Domain 2)

1. A decline in the unemployment rate that typically accompanies a period of economic expansion makes recruiting new employees even tougher because _____.

   A. Wages are depressed
   B. Fewer people are available or looking or work
   C. Recruiting expenses become cost-prohibitive
   D. Senior living pays less than unemployment insurance benefits

2. In screening employment applications, ranking each résumé by the extent to which it aligns with the position specifications is called _____.

   A. Parsing
   B. Collating
   C. Sifting
   D. Filtering

3. Which of the following is not a key benefit of requiring a prospective employee to apply in person?

   A. Observe the applicant's reading and writing proficiency
   B. Ensure the application is complete
   C. Determine "fit" with the organization's culture
   D. Meet the applicant

4. Which is the most cost-effective preemployment drug test?

   A. Six-panel blood assay
   B. Eight-panel hair follicle test
   C. Seven-panel saliva test
   D. Five-panel urinalysis test

5. The most critical limitation of maintaining a "zero-tolerance" policy concerning an employee testing positive for the active agent in marijuana, tetrahydrocannabinol (THC), is the _____.

   A. Change in contemporary social norms
   B. Importance of protecting non-work-related personal privacy
   C. Inconsistent reliability of available tests
   D. Lack of scientific evidence of an amount that causes impairment

6. When an organization responds to a reference request concerning a former employee by providing only their dates of tenure, it is most likely _____.
   A. Minimizing its own liability risk
   B. Hinting there may be a problem
   C. Hoping the employee will return
   D. Striving for consistency in reference reporting

7. Constructing an effective professional development plan (PDP) begins with _____.
   A. Assessing a person's current knowledge, skills, and interests
   B. Evaluating the organization's needs for expertise and skill sets
   C. Exploring internal professional advancement opportunities
   D. Comparing the internal career ladder with external opportunities

8. An employee's professional development plan should ideally _____.
   A. Exceed those of the person they replace
   B. Align their aspirations and interests with the opportunities available within the field
   C. Align their aspirations and interests with the opportunities available within the organization
   D. Include stretch goals for continuous growth

9. A structured sequence of positions through which a person can advance reflecting greater scope of responsibility, professional competencies, and/or pay is commonly referred to as a _____.
   A. Professional growth tract
   B. Career ladder
   C. Vocational progression pathway
   D. Skill set enhancement plan

10. The most effective performance appraisal formats provide meaningful feedback to an employee that reward them for meeting or exceeding expectations and _____.
    A. Enable scheduling flexibility
    B. Publicly honor achievement
    C. Identify opportunities for growth and improvement
    D. Offer a cost-of-living adjustment

11. Contemporary leaders find that replacing traditional supervisory techniques with ongoing _____ interventions gets better results concerning productivity, employee engagement, and retention.
    A. Management by walking around
    B. Coaching
    C. Emotional intelligence
    D. Training

12. An organization's compensation strategy is considered _____ when it strives to consistently land at a targeted goal in comparison with the wages paid for similar jobs among its peers.
    A. Aspirational
    B. Market driven
    C. Competition centric
    D. Environment conscious

13. A _____ compensation strategy calls for determining pay ranges based on the availability of qualified workers in a particular location and the intensity of competition for those people among area employers.
    A. Growth-oriented
    B. Open-ended
    C. Competition-based
    D. Market-driven

14. A fringe benefit—an incidental payment, privilege, or advantage over and above regular wages—is sometimes called a _____.
    A. Bonus
    B. Perk
    C. Incentive
    D. Gratuity

15. Short-term disability insurance typically provides benefits that replace _____ of a full-time employee's normal gross wages.
    A. 60%–75%
    B. 50%–55%
    C. 80%–90%
    D. 35%–45%

16. To qualify for receiving benefits under a long-term disability insurance plan, an employee is generally required to first be continuously disabled for at least _____ months.
    A. 9
    B. 6
    C. 3
    D. 12

17. The U.S. Internal Revenue Code allows for providing as a fringe benefit up to $_____ in group term life insurance benefits without affecting an employee's taxable income.
    A. 75,000
    B. 10,000
    C. 25,000
    D. 50,000

18. Workers' compensation insurance in most states provides at least the following basic benefits for a staff member injured on the job: medical care, temporary and permanent disability coverage, death benefits to their family if caused by a work-related injury, and _____.
    A. A disabled parking permit
    B. Vocational retraining
    C. Job displacement services
    D. Housing subsidy assistance

19. The government agency that sets minimum standards for determining who qualifies for unemployment insurance (UI) benefits is the _____.
    A. U.S. Department of Labor
    B. State Insurance Department
    C. Local Unemployment Office
    D. Fair Labor Standards Board

20. The most familiar qualified employee benefit plans are profit-sharing and stock option programs, both of which are governed by the _____.
    A. Title XX of the Social Security Act
    B. Employee Retirement Income Security Act
    C. Fair Labor Standards Act
    D. Federal Employee Benefits Improvement Act

21. A _____ retirement plan incentivizes saving for retirement by deferring income taxes on the earnings deposited by an individual in a special account for this purpose.
    A. Defined contribution
    B. Postponed liability
    C. Deliberate annuity
    D. Defined benefit

22. A health savings account (HSA) reduces an employee's out-of-pocket costs, lowers their income tax liability, rolls over from year to year, and _____.
    A. Is exempt from bank management fees
    B. Lowers an employer's payroll taxes
    C. Can be transferred to another employee of the same organization
    D. Varies by state

23. According to the U.S. Bureau of Department of Labor's Bureau of Labor Statistics, _____ of American employees receive paid time off from work for either sick or vacation time.
    A. Nearly 90%
    B. Between 60% and 70%
    C. Over 75%
    D. Under 50%

24. As employee engagement goes up, organizations typically experience greater productivity and lower rates of turnover, absenteeism, tardiness, work injuries, conflicts, and _____.
    A. Grievances
    B. Rehospitalizations
    C. Terminations
    D. Illness

25. The Wagner Act created an independent federal agency that protects the rights of private sector employees to join together to form and join a union, known as the _____.
    A. U.S. Department of Labor
    B. National Labor Relations Board
    C. U.S. Bureau of Labor Statistics
    D. Federal Wage and Hour Division

26. Effectively establishing and building a workplace culture that fosters professional and personal growth, engagement, fulfillment, and favorable outcomes for the organization and for those served by it takes a leader who consistently demonstrates vision, empathy and compassion, discernment, integrity, _____, and stamina.
    A. Command
    B. Presence
    C. Transparency
    D. Insight

27. In order to maintain an organizational culture that nurtures professional and personal growth, fosters engagement and fulfillment, and produces favorable outcomes for those it serves, a health services executive must recognize the potential each person brings to the table and demonstrate a sincere willingness to invest in their _____ development.
    A. Short-term and lifelong
    B. Academic and vocational
    C. Career plan
    D. Professional and personal

28. A workplace culture that encourages professional and personal growth, interdependent engagement, life fulfillment, and favorable outcomes for the organization's customers and other stakeholders requires a leader who can master the art of nurturing _____ and _____ relationships.
    A. Staff, family
    B. Customer, community
    C. New, long-standing
    D. Complex, multidirectional

29. In healthcare, the most common jurisdiction for enforcing adherence to professional standards are _____ boards of licensure.
    A. National
    B. Local
    C. State
    D. Accredited

30. The most important motivational aspect of work for most people is _____.
    A. Understanding opportunities for advancement
    B. Personal time and attention by one's supervisor
    C. Equitable wages and benefits
    D. Job security

31. The most actionable contributing factor to absenteeism for leadership to address is an employee missing work due to _____.
    A. Slippery onboarding
    B. Transportation
    C. Illness
    D. Exhaustion

32. Over one in _____ American workers admit to being tardy at least once a month, and _____% are late once a week, or more.
    A. Four, 16
    B. Three, 20
    C. Five, 25
    D. Six, 15

33. Whether it is for an organization's current operations or for envisioning a strategic direction for the future, _____ is essential to success and a hallmark of effective leadership.
    A. Budgeting
    B. Listening
    C. Planning
    D. Communication

34. Business author and Stanford University professor Jim Collins, in his book *Good to Great*, suggests that the most effective leaders continuously ask, _____
    A. "How does this support the mission?"
    B. "How do we begin with the end in mind?"
    C. "First who, then what?"
    D. "Do those I serve grow as persons?"

35. Equipping people with the knowledge and skills to perform assignments outside of the realm of their normal position to add flexibility and bench strength for the operation is called _____.
    A. Flex scheduling
    B. A career ladder
    C. Horizontal development
    D. Cross-training

36. An effective health services executive not only oversees employee performance but also instructs, guides, and inspires—_____—the growth and development of each member of the work team in order to most effectively and efficiently achieve desired goals and objectives.
    A. Commands
    B. Coaches
    C. Supports
    D. Orchestrates

37. "Direction" in leadership typically has the following characteristics: pervasive function, continuous activity, human factor, creative activity, and the _____ function.
    A. Delegate
    B. Accountability
    C. Disciplinary
    D. Counseling

38. One can delegate _____ but not _____.
    A. Assignments, strategic goals
    B. Authority, responsibility
    C. Responsibility, authority
    D. Tasks, authority

39. People who feel consistently rewarded and find their work _____ tend to stay with the organization longer, and they are typically more _____ because of their familiarity with the duties of the job and with the needs and preferences of the clients.
    A. Challenging, efficient
    B. Easy, loyal
    C. Fulfilling, productive
    D. Rewarding, reliable

40. Which of the following is *not* considered among the top workplace motivators?
    A. Control or influence
    B. Cafeteria plan benefits
    C. Insider membership
    D. Growth and development

41. Employees are typically more highly motivated when they feel they can count on their leader to do the following: convey their vision for the future and its alignment with the organization's mission and values; show respect, transparency, and sincerity; and consistently _____.
    A. Apply fair and equal treatment
    B. Pay the highest wage in the market
    C. Remember their name
    D. Circulate among employees

42. The reputation of a health services executive as a trustworthy leader who is deserving of people's loyalty ties closely to how well they are perceived as someone who consistently _____.
    A. Mentors those with the most promise
    B. Respects every person's confidentiality
    C. Fights for higher wages in the budget
    D. Works longer hours than anyone else

43. High-performing work teams typically require both good leadership and _____—and that each member recognizes when it is best to engage in either.
    A. Followership
    B. Competitors
    C. Diversity
    D. Metrics

44. Embracing the value of diversity as a strength-building characteristic of an organization is an effective way to demonstrate _____.
    A. Sympathy
    B. Empathy
    C. Wisdom
    D. Respect

45. In addition to the blend of races, genders and identity, religions, and national origins, the notion of inclusiveness also has implications for shared governance, employee empowerment, balance of perspectives, and _____.
    A. Depth of engagement
    B. Equal Employment Opportunity Commission compliance
    C. Cost-effectiveness
    D. Customer satisfaction

ANSWERS AND RATIONALES

1. Answer: **B.** When job vacancies outpace the number of people available to fill them, job recruiters have fewer choices.

2. Answer: **A.** Résumé parsing is more than organizing or arranging applications; it involves analyzing content and aligning qualifications with position requirements.

3. Answer: **C.** Applying in person does not necessarily entail an interview or exchange that would provide a basis for determining alignment with the organization's culture.

4. Answer: **D.** The U.S. Department of Transportation utilizes this test for hiring people in safety-sensitive positions and considers it the most cost-effective preemployment drug test available.

5. Answer: **D.** Impairment in response to THC varies widely by a person's body type, body mass index, and underlying health conditions; there is not yet an established level of THC that accurately predicts one's ability to perform job tasks.

6. Answer: **A.** An effective way to avoid a legal action by a former, underperforming employee who lists the organization as a reference is to limit information shared about *any* former employee to facts.

7. Answer: **A.** Just as "person-centered care" focuses on the customer, a PDP is most useful if a purposeful plan aimed at growth in areas that need developing first identifies those opportunities.

8. Answer: **C.** An organization is often more inclined to invest in a person's growth and development when there is a reasonable prospect of that contributing to the advancement of its mission.

9. Answer: **B.** The ladder metaphor depicts rising in one's career and is widely used to convey the notion of climbing higher and higher from one's current position.

10. Answer: **C.** People want to know that there is a brighter future available and what needs to happen for it to happen.

11. Answer: **B.** Coaching involves mentoring, teaching, and motivating someone; the alternate response options are each tools that can prove useful for coaching.

12. Answer: **A.** "Aspirational" means meeting a goal or target.

13. Answer: **D.** "Market-driven" strategy is a derivative of the economic laws of supply and demand.

14. Answer: **B.** *Perk* is short for *perquisite*, a special right or privilege enjoyed as a result of one's position.

15. Answer: **A.** Short-term disability plans pay benefits based on an employee's pretax income—generally about two thirds.

16. Answer: **B.** Long-term disability plans are typically designed to trigger when an employee remains disabled after a significant qualifying period of at least 6 months.

17. Answer: **D.** The answer follows per IRS Publication 15-B found at www.irs .gov/pub/irs-pdf/p15b.pdf.

18. Answer: **C.** None of the alternate response options are typically included in a state's core workers' compensation benefit plan.

19. Answer: **A.** Federal law establishes that the U.S. Department of Labor set minimum standards that states governments must meet for UI benefits.

20. Answer: **B.** They have the same rules for eligibility, allocation of benefits, and vesting, and contributions to either are tax deductible. Title XX of the Social Security Act provides for funding for social services through the Social Services Block Grant program; the Fair Labor Standards Act governs union organizing and fair labor practices; the Federal Employees Benefits Improvement Act of 1986 addresses benefits for federal employees.

21. Answer: **A.** One typically pays taxes at a lower rate when retired, so the amount contributed through many years grows with interest compounding but has greater buying power after taxes are applied in later years at a lower rate.

22. Answer: **B.** HSA contributions reduce the amount of employee wages on which an employer's payroll taxes are based.

23. Answer: **C.** See www.bls.gov.

24. Answer: **A.** The highest correlation with employee engagement is a reduction in grievances filed by staff.

25. Answer: **B.** Also known as the National Labor Relations Act of 1935, the Wagner Act guarantees the right of private sector employees to organize into trade unions, engage in collective bargaining, and take collective actions, such as strikes.

26. Answer: **C.** Transparency breeds trust and loyalty.

27. Answer: **D.** Genuine interest in the whole person—professional and private—fosters this kind of organizational culture.

28. Answer: **D.** Senior living leadership demands more than intellect; it requires emotional intelligence to manage the complexity and speed of business.

29. Answer: **C.** Licensing of healthcare professionals is considered a states' rights issue.

30. Answer: **B.** Answer is supported in the following: American Psychological Association. (2014). *Employee recognition survey.* www.apaexcellence.org/assets/general/employee-recognition-survey-results.pdf

31. Answer: **A.** An employee who is less confident about what is expected and about how to perform the duties of the position is more likely to come late, leave early, or miss work in order to cope with the uncertainty.

32. Answer: **A.** Answer is supported in the following: Smith, J. (2013, February 8). The most ridiculous excuses from tardy employees. *Forbes.* www.forbes.com/sites/jacquelynsmith/2013/02/08/the-most-ridiculous-excuses-from-tardy-employees/

33. Answer: **C.** Setting the course for the organization—short or long term—is an absolutely critical duty of its leader.

34. Answer: **C.** Answer is supported in the following: Collins, J. (2001). *Good to great: Why some companies make the leap and others don't.* HarperCollins Publishing (p. 44).

35. Answer: **D.** A properly cross-trained staff member enables management to assign duties in multiple areas on differing days based on the organization's changing needs.

36. Answer: **B.** Coaching involves all of the elements listed.

37. Answer: **A.** Each of the alternate response options falls into another category of management and leadership—monitoring.

38. Answer: **B.** Authority is the power to act; responsibility is the duty to act.

39. Answer: **C.** Job fulfillment and productivity are highly correlated.

40. Answer: **B.** Job fulfillment and productivity are highly correlated.

41. Answer: **A.** People highly value justice, fairness, and consistency.

42. Answer: **B.** Trust is paramount for a leader to earn and maintain, and it starts with preserving confidentiality.

43. Answer: **A.** Not every person on a team can serve as its leader all the time. It takes willing followers to embrace the direction set by the leader for the team to succeed.

44. Answer: **D.** It is not enough to be tolerant of people with other views, backgrounds, traditions, or cultures. Proactively demonstrating commitment to inclusion and diversity affirms one's respect for all.

45. Answer: **A.** People are often more inclined to engage with more intensity and consistency when they feel truly included in a diverse workforce.

CHAPTER 4

Financial Management in Senior Care (NAB Domain 3)

1. The amount of money spent on medical supplies in a particular month would appear on which financial report?
   A. Income statement
   B. Balance sheet
   C. Cash flow statement
   D. Operating budget

2. The reimbursed expenses for travel related to continuing education annually are shown on which financial report?
   A. Balance sheet
   B. Cash flow statement
   C. Operating budget
   D. Income statement

3. The amount of money invested in short-term financial instruments is reported in an organization's _____.
   A. Income statement
   B. Cash flow statement
   C. Balance sheet
   D. Operating budget

4. The total of accounts receivable—money owed to the organization for services already performed—is reported in which financial report?
   A. Balance sheet
   B. Income statement
   C. Cash flow statement
   D. Operating budget

5. The three main categories of financial metrics used for business operations monitoring measure an organization's capital position, profitability, and _____.
   A. Risk exposure
   B. Liquidity
   C. Speed of business
   D. Stability

6. An operating margin ratio is calculated by _____.
   A. Dividing current assets by current liabilities
   B. Adding depreciation to net operating income and dividing by resident days
   C. Dividing cash and cash equivalents by operating expenses less depreciation and then dividing by 365 days
   D. Subtracting expenses from revenues and then dividing by revenues

7. Liquidity ratios reflect the ability of an organization to _____.
   A. Weather a severe economic downturn
   B. Cover its current liabilities
   C. Invest in capital expansion
   D. Attract investors

8. Which of the following is considered a measure of an organization's liquidity?
   A. Debt service coverage
   B. Current ratio
   C. Net operating ratio
   D. Bond rating

9. The quotient resulting from dividing an organization's current assets by its current liabilities is known as its _____ ratio.
   A. Acid test
   B. Capital
   C. Current
   D. Liquidity

10. The _____ ratio reflects commitment to reinvestment, and it is calculated by dividing the annual capital spending by total revenues.
    A. Capital spending
    B. Debt to capitalization
    C. Net operating
    D. Acid test

11. The chief financial officer (CFO) oversees the fiscal support functions, such as management of accounts payable, payroll, cash flow, budgeting, financial performance monitoring and reporting, bank reconciliations and relationships, purchasing, resident funds, and _____.
    A. Utilities consumption
    B. Inventory control
    C. Accounts receivable
    D. Corporate compliance

12. One of the biggest expenses in all senior care services is the costs associated with labor, including basic wages and overtime pay, paid time off, temporary supplemental staff, training, and _____.
    A. Employer payroll taxes
    B. Health insurance
    C. Uniforms
    D. Transportation

13. An operating budget includes both variable and _____ expenses.
    A. Flexible
    B. Time-limited
    C. Fixed
    D. Unanticipated

14. Capital budgeting is planning for large purchases that _____.
    A. Replace assets reaching the end of their useful lives
    B. Expand building capacity or equipment capability
    C. Require an accompanying maintenance contract
    D. Have a useful life of over a year

15. Which of the following items would likely appear in a capital budget?
    A. One-year supply of paper towels
    B. Telephone system
    C. Lawn care contract
    D. Vehicle lease

16. Borrowing money and repaying the principal with interest is a form of capital acquisition known as _____ financing.
    A. Equity
    B. Risk
    C. Debt
    D. Loan

17. _____ financing calls for capital sources to invest in an organization in exchange for part ownership.
    A. Debt
    B. Partnership
    C. Stakeholder
    D. Equity

18. Bonds can have either a fixed or _____ interest rate.
    A. A variable
    B. A commercial
    C. A prime
    D. A capped

19. An ownership structure that combines the characteristics of a corporation with those of a partnership or sole proprietorship, in which the owners are not personally liable for the company's debts or liabilities, is known as a/an _____.
    A. Real estate investment trust
    B. Multilevel marketing corporation
    C. Limited liability corporation (LLC)
    D. Employee stock ownership plan

20. A/an _____ is composed of a pool of investor dollars used to acquire healthcare real estate assets.
    A. Employee stock ownership plan
    B. Real estate investment trust (REIT)
    C. Limited liability corporation
    D. Blind pool investment fund

21. A health services executive (HSE™) needs to be committed to the needs of the organization, visible, visionary, and personally involved in _____.
    A. Capital development efforts
    B. Resident trust fund monitoring
    C. Civic and community organizations
    D. Developing cash flow projections

22. Which of the following is the least common source of capital among government-sponsored senior living organizations?
    A. U.S. Department of Agriculture
    B. Department of Housing and Urban Development
    C. Real estate investment trust (REIT)
    D. Federal Housing Administration

23. The REIT Investment, Diversification, and Empowerment Act of 2007 allows real estate investment trusts (REITs) to use a/an _____ structure to keep a share of the building's operating income and not just the lease payments.
    A. Partnership
    B. S corporation
    C. Proprietary
    D. Not-for-profit

24. State Medicaid programs most commonly support the provision of home- and community-based services through waivers available under the Social Security Act's section 1915(b) or _____.
    A. 1199
    B. The Older Americans Act (OAA)
    C. 1915(c)
    D. Title XVIII

25. The formula for determining each state's financial contribution to fund its Medicaid program and the complementary federal share relies on the state's _____ relative to all the other states.
    A. Percentage of eligible citizens
    B. Per capita federal tax burden
    C. Number of eligible people
    D. Per capita income

26. A private insurance plan purchased as a method to pay for expenses not covered by Medicare must be identified as a _____ plan to be valid.
    A. Medicare Supplement Insurance
    B. Medi-Guard
    C. Part C
    D. Long-Term Care Partnership

27. Medicare accounts for _____ of the reimbursement received by home health and hospice providers.
    A. Greater than two thirds
    B. Over 40%
    C. Under 25%
    D. About one half

28. A free market system in which temporary positions are common and organizations contract with independent workers for short-term engagements is known as a _____ economy.
    A. Gig
    B. Supply
    C. Demand
    D. Flex

29. Research suggests that to attract the best employees, an organization should expect to pay _____ its _____ counterparts in the marketplace.
    A. Less than, highest-paying
    B. More than, average-paying
    C. About the same as, closest local
    D. Better than, service industry

30. A person's payment source has the most significant influence on access to which of the following senior living lines of service?
    A. Skilled nursing facility
    B. Hospice
    C. Medicaid waiver home health
    D. Adult day care

ANSWERS AND RATIONALES

1. Answer: **A.** According to generally accepted accounting principles, which are set forth by the Financial Accounting Standards Board, this expense happens in the current accounting period.

2. Answer: **D.** According to generally accepted accounting principles, which are set forth by the Financial Accounting Standards Board, this expense happens in the current accounting period.

3. Answer: **C.** According to generally accepted accounting principles, which are set forth by the Financial Accounting Standards Board, this money is considered a current asset.

4. Answer: **A.** According to generally accepted accounting principles, which are set forth by the Financial Accounting Standards Board, the amount owed has been earned, but not collected yet.

5. Answer: **B.** Liquidity refers to how easily assets can be converted into cash, usually measured by subtracting current liabilities from current assets.

6. Answer: **D.** The operating margin ratio illustrates the relationship between profit (margin) and revenues.

7. Answer: **B.** A positive liquidity ratio indicates that the organization owns enough liquid assets to convert them to cash and pay all of its obligations—with some leftover.

8. Answer: **B.** The current ratio is a liquidity ratio that shows how an organization can maximize the current assets on its balance sheet to satisfy its current debt and other payables.

9. Answer: **C.** The current ratio is a liquidity ratio that shows how an organization can maximize the value of its current assets (numerator) to satisfy its current liabilities (denominator).

10. Answer: **A.** Also known as Cap/Ex Ratio, this reflects the organization's ability to finance its own capital needs at the expense of the operating activity.

11. Answer: **C.** Accounts receivable (a.k.a. A/R)—the money owed to the organization for services rendered—is a primary responsibility of the CFO.

12. Answer: **A.** All employers have payroll taxes; not all offer health insurance, provide uniforms, or subsidize transportation.

13. Answer: **C.** Variable expenses are tied to fluctuations in census, revenues, or expenses (such as staffing or supplies), and fixed expenses typically remain constant (such as a mortgage).

14. Answer: **D.** One feature of a "capital" asset is that it typically lasts longer than 1 year, so the cost of its purchase is generally spread across its anticipated useful life.

15. Answer: **B.** A capital purchase is a large amount (an organization determines the threshold, typically $1,000–5,000), and it acquires an asset with a useful life of more than 1 year.

16. Answer: **C.** Paying for a capital expense over time often requires incurring debt, which typically requires the borrower to repay both the loan principal and interest.

17. Answer: **D.** When the lender takes an ownership interest in the enterprise, the lender gains an "equity position" that allows it a share in any net proceeds from the future sale of the company.

18. Answer: **A.** A variable interest rate means that it can be adjusted according to the terms agreed to in the loan documents, sometimes with limits governing how much it is permitted to change.

19. Answer: **C.** The adjective "limited" reflects the key difference between an LLC and either a partnership or a sole proprietorship.

20. Answer: **B.** REIT-owned healthcare properties offer an alternative to conventional bank loans or bonds but typically charge a slightly higher interest rate in exchange for ease of access to funds needed for a provider to expand and modernize its physical plant.

21. Answer: **A.** Capital needed for modernization or expansion is typically identified and integrated into the organization's strategic plan; as the "community face" for the organization, the HSE™ must play an active role in securing the resources necessary for supporting the strategic direction.

22. Answer: **C.** Many more providers access grants and loans from federal sources for capital expenditures—particularly construction—than private REITs.

23. Answer: **A.** Instead of just underwriting a steady rent payment and annual escalation, REITs can analyze and underwrite larger shifts in operations and income through the vehicle of a partnership.

24. Answer: **C.** Medicaid = Title XVIII of the Social Security Act. The OAA is not part of the Social Security Act; "1199" typically refers to District 1199—the Services Employees International Union.

25. Answer: **D.** The collective wealth of a state's citizens—relative to that of all other states—is the chief determinant of how federal funds earmarked for Medicaid programs are distributed.

26. Answer: **A.** Federal law requires this descriptive title.

27. Answer: **B.** According to the Centers for Medicare & Medicaid Services, more than 40% of revenues received by home health agencies and hospice providers come from Medicare.

28. Answer: **A.** The phrase "gig economy" was coined at the height of the financial crisis in early 2009, when many unemployed people made a living by gigging, or working several part-time jobs, wherever they could (derived from musicians playing at multiple, unrelated venues).

29. Answer: **B.** Answer is supported in the following: Pfau, B. N., & Kay, I. T. (2001). *The human capital edge: 21 people management practices your company must implement (or avoid) to maximize shareholder value.* McGraw-Hill.

30. Answer: **C.** Each alternate response option describes a service line that can accept other sources of payment than Medicaid, which is a means-tested program.

CHAPTER 5

Environment (NAB Domain 4)

1. Most states, and even some local governments, have established building and construction codes with the fundamental purpose of _____.
   A. Public protection
   B. Zoning consistency
   C. Generating nontax revenues
   D. Extending the useful life of buildings

2. The _____ is/are the premier source for strategies to protect people based on building construction, protection, and occupancy features that minimize the effects of fire and related hazards.
   A. Contemporary Building Standards Code
   B. American Institute of Architects Design Guidelines
   C. Life Safety Code (National Fire Protection Association-101 [NFPA]-101)
   D. NCBCS Whole Building Design Guide

3. Finding the optimal blend of internal effort and purchased services for groundskeeping requires _____.
   A. Competitive bidding
   B. Ongoing evaluation
   C. Broadly trained staff
   D. Flexible scheduling

4. In a senior living setting, "security" typically concerns _____.
   A. Perimeter protection or containment
   B. Elopement or theft prevention
   C. Surveillance or infection control
   D. Safe access and egress

5. A disaster preparedness plan must consider all plausible hazards, define operations during the disaster (including communication and coordination with other healthcare providers and the community), include a training and drilling component, and undergo internal review at least _____.
   A. Semiannually
   B. Biannually
   C. Quarterly
   D. Annually

6. A hazard vulnerability analysis includes detailed descriptions of the organization's incident command division of responsibilities, response plan, communication tactics for keeping stakeholders informed, and _____.
   A. Training and drills
   B. Sources and uses of financial support
   C. Alternate transportation methods
   D. Just-in-time inventory control

7. An emergency or disaster that affects only one part of a building may require a/an _____, which is transferring residents to another section of the same building or to an adjacent structure in order to preserve their safety.
   A. Cross-facility cohorting
   B. Complete evacuation
   C. Partial evacuation
   D. Internal transfer

8. In the senior living field, the acronym GPO most commonly refers to_____.
   A. Gross production output
   B. General personnel outlook
   C. Group purchasing organization
   D. Geriatric practitioner organization

9. An effective price analysis process includes developing product specifications that objectively address _____, composition, availability, weight, and size.
   A. Packaging
   B. Price
   C. Distribution
   D. Quality grade

10. _____ is the term applied to describe the procedures regarding where to physically accept delivery of goods that were ordered, stock the inventory, and verify that the invoice matches the packing sheet with respect to units delivered and product specifications and that prices charged reflect the prices in the current contract.
    A. Receiving
    B. Verification
    C. Cross-checking
    D. Delivery

11. Rotating stocked items in such a fashion that the newest arrivals are stored for last retrieval reflects an accounting principle called _____.
    A. Stock rotation
    B. First-in first-out (FIFO)
    C. Last-in first-out
    D. Inventory sequencing

12. A _____ level is the amount of a product that is typically needed to meet the residents' collective needs for any restocking cycle—per shift, day, week, or month.
    A. PAR
    B. Demand
    C. Period
    D. Stock

13. Information that should be prominently and legibly displayed on a container that has been opened and stored, as well as food that has been prepared and saved for future serving, includes date, time, _____, and the name of the person completing the label.
    A. When to use by or dispose
    B. Reheating temperature
    C. Replacement order date
    D. Contents

14. An organization's governing body, a group of people who accept legal responsibility for how the organization operates and who oversee its performance, is most commonly referred to as the organization's _____.
    A. Fiduciary trust
    B. Board of directors
    C. Moral compass
    D. Stakeholder system

15. A highly effective health services executive equips the organization's governing board by regularly supplying and interpreting _____.
    A. Internal and external reports
    B. Industry trends
    C. Inspection reports
    D. Media coverage

16. Reports by executive leadership to the governing board on external forces that have the potential to affect the operation commonly include challenges and opportunities tied to decisions made by competing providers, proposed or recently approved legislation or regulations, innovations and professional trends in the field, or _____ that may impact the operation.
    A. Shifts in case mix distribution
    B. Vacant positions
    C. Economic developments
    D. Staff retention rate

17. The four elements to incorporate into a governing board's dashboard or balanced scorecard are the perspectives of the customer, internal operations, financial stakeholders, and _____.
    A. The staff
    B. The environment
    C. Innovation and learning
    D. Regulatory compliance

18. A balanced scorecard for a senior living organization would likely address its goals and metrics for staff development or technology as part of the _____ perspective.
    A. Innovation and learning
    B. Customer
    C. Financial
    D. Internal operations

19. A balanced scorecard for a senior living organization would likely address its goals and metrics for person-centered care and quality services as part of the _____ perspective.
    A. Innovation and learning
    B. Customer
    C. Financial
    D. Internal operations

20. The chief limitation of a public policy that sets the standard for regulatory compliance in senior living settings at meeting minimal standards is that this approach _____.
    A. Is subject to budgetary restrictions
    B. Requires uniform interpretation
    C. Measures capacity instead of outcomes
    D. Lacks incentives for achieving excellence

21. Individual states reserve the right to govern the practice of health professionals through discipline-specific professional practice acts, the primary purpose of which is _____.
    A. Public protection
    B. Practice standardization
    C. Enforcing guidelines
    D. Disciplinary action

22. The nation's oldest and largest healthcare standards–setting and accrediting body, which evaluates and accredits over 21,000 health providers, from hospitals to skilled nursing facilities, home health agencies, and hospices, is known as the _____.
    A. Centers for Medicare & Medicaid Services
    B. Blue Cross and Blue Shield Federation
    C. Joint Commission
    D. International Organization for Standards

23. _____ laws deal with the legal punishment of behavior that is an offense against the public, society, or the state, such as theft or murder.
    A. Criminal
    B. Civil
    C. Tort
    D. Constitutional

24. In a civil suit, the entity initiating the legal action is called the _____, and the entity charged with harming the plaintiff is called the _____.
    A. Attorney-in-fact, defendant
    B. Plaintiff, defendant
    C. Plaintiff, accused
    D. Complainant, suspect

25. If a contract promise is breached, the law provides remedies to the harmed party, often in the form of monetary damages, or in limited circumstances, in the form of _____.
    A. Specific performance of the promise made
    B. Remuneration and court costs
    C. Incarceration
    D. Community service

26. In _____, the disputing parties decide whether to agree to a settlement; the _____ they jointly select has no power to impose a binding resolution. In _____, the parties assign authority to decide the dispute to a jointly selected _____.
    A. Arbitration, arbitrator, mediation, mediator
    B. Mediation, mediator, arbitration, hearing officer
    C. Mediation, mediator, arbitration, arbitrator
    D. Arbitration, judge, mediation, mediator

27. When a provider ignores or fails to take reasonable measures to prevent harm from happening to a care recipient in its charge, it may result in a claim of _____.
    A. Assault
    B. Battery
    C. False imprisonment
    D. Negligence

28. _____ are among the most commonly cited reasons for people to move from their homes to a congregate living setting and highly rated as concerns for those who remain at home with contracted supports and services.
    A. Safety and security
    B. Transportation and healthcare access
    C. Loneliness and helplessness
    D. Grief and loss

29. _____ is a process that systematically surveys and interprets relevant data to identify external opportunities and threats by gathering information about the external world, its competitors, and itself.
    A. Relevant benchmarking
    B. Environmental scanning
    C. Redundant probing
    D. Climate checking

30. Supports and services that are emphasized in the home- and community-based services (HCBS) realm include emergency security alert systems, home modification and installing "smart home" devices, professional geriatric care management, and _____.
    A. Certified nursing assistant training
    B. Disaster preparedness planning
    C. Virtual/online visitation
    D. Transportation

ANSWERS AND RATIONALES

1. Answer: **A.** The overriding objective of construction standards is protecting the public from dangers posed by improperly designed or built structures and public spaces.

2. Answer: **C.** The NFPA publishes evidence-based standards for this purpose: the NFPA-101.

3. Answer: **B.** Productivity and cost-effectiveness can change over time, so monitoring the cost–benefit of the current mix of internal and outsourced service delivery is important.

4. Answer: **A.** Keeping unwanted, unauthorized visitors from entering and guarding against unplanned or contraindicated departures by residents is the essential goal of providing security in senior living settings.

5. Answer: **D.** The Centers for Medicare & Medicaid Services requires a disaster preparedness plan to be reviewed at least annually.

6. Answer: **A.** Practicing the planned response is key to achieving success in the event of an actual disaster event.

7. Answer: **C.** A partial evacuation can result in safely situating people—residents and staff—without emptying the entire building in certain circumstances.

8. Answer: **C.** Pooling the purchasing power of two or more providers—leveraging the volume of goods and services needed to drive discounting of prices—can be achieved through a group purchasing organization.

9. Answer: **D.** Quality grade is the only response option that is a product specification.

10. Answer: **A.** The organization "receives" the goods it has ordered when delivered.

11. Answer: **B.** FIFO reduces the risk of an item with an expiration date to wait too long in inventory by sitting at the rear.

12. Answer: **A.** PAR stands for *periodic automatic replenishment* (average inventory usage + safety stock)/(number of deliveries per time period).

13. Answer: **D.** Describing accurately what is inside a container prevents opening it to find out—and exposing the contents to air—as well as using the contents by mistake.

14. Answer: **B.** A corporate governing body "directs" and sets the mission, values, and vision for its future.

15. Answer: **A.** In order for the governing board to make informed decisions, it must have current, accurate, and complete data about the internal operation, as well as about community and industry trends that can influence those decisions.

16. Answer: **C.** Each of the alternate response options is the report on an internal phenomenon.

17. Answer: **C.** The concept of a balanced scorecard was introduced by Kaplan and Norton in 1992. This performance measurement approach has since been widely adopted as a high-impact practice among businesses in many industries, and allows managers to look at their organizations from four different perspectives. Kaplan, R. S., & Norton, D. P. (1992, January/February). The balanced scorecard—Measures that drive performance. *Harvard Business Review*. hbr.org/1992/01/the-balanced -scorecard-measures-that-drive-performance-2

18. Answer: **A.** The concept of a balanced scorecard (Kaplan and Norton, 1992) advocates that staff development and technology most closely pertain to innovation and learning.

19. Answer: **B.** The concept of a balanced scorecard (Kaplan and Norton, 1992) suggests the person-centered experience and quality of services (as perceived by the recipient) most closely align with the customer perspective.

20. Answer: **D.** Monitoring and enforcing compliance with minimal standards sets a relatively low bar and fails to reward high-performing providers.

21. Answer: **A.** Licensing of health professionals is considered a protected state's right (not a federal right).

22. Answer: **C.** It was originally known as the Joint Commission on Accreditation of Hospitals and then the Joint Commission on Accreditation of Health Care Organizations; it is now simply The Joint Commission.

23. Answer: **A.** A criminal offense (crime) is a type of wrongdoing that is viewed as harming not only the specific victim but also the sensibilities of society as a whole.

24. Answer: **B.** The plaintiff claims (complaint) wrongdoing by the defendant (who defends against the complaint).

25. Answer: **A.** One available remedy for a breach of contract is to require the defendant to partially or completely fulfill the terms of the contract.

26. Answer: **C.** A mediator referees negotiations between parties to find a mutually agreeable resolution through mediation; an arbitrator acts as a judge to determine the outcome.

27. Answer: **D.** Negligence is an act of omission—failure to do something for which there is a duty—and it causes harm; the other response options are each acts of commission—intentional actions that result in harm.

28. Answer: **A.** Whether self-assessed or evaluated by others, safety and security are highly valued by those who experience difficulty in continuing to provide either for themselves.

29. Answer: **B.** Remaining constantly aware of changes internally and in the surrounding business and regulatory environment is critical to adapt successfully.

30. Answer: **D.** Transportation provides an essential lifeline in the HCBS arena for both care recipients and care providers.

CHAPTER 6

Management and Leadership: Providing a Context (NAB Domain 5)

1. The _____ view of leadership is used to identify formal positions of authority.
   A. Hierarchical
   B. Shared influence
   C. Specialized role
   D. Vertical distribution

2. The informal influence that seems to naturally occur in any kind of social group by anyone at any time is called the _____ view of leadership.
   A. Shared influence
   B. Vertical distribution
   C. Specialized role
   D. Spontaneous generation

3. A common link found among most research on leadership is that it involves _____ influence in a group or organization.
   A. Powerful
   B. Consistent
   C. Proactive
   D. Purposeful

4. It is the _____ rather than the _____ of leadership and management that are distinct, and they do not necessarily require different types of people.
   A. Processes, roles
   B. Roles, functions
   C. Roles, processes
   D. Authority, responsibility

5. An unbalanced focus on _____ processes may discourage innovation and risk-taking while producing a bureaucracy without clear purpose.
   A. Supervisory
   B. Management
   C. Leadership
   D. Quality assurance and performance improvement

6. Management is generally associated with _____.
   A. Looking to the future of the organization
   B. Change
   C. Day-to-day operations
   D. Preserving traditions

7. Leadership is generally associated with _____.
   A. Working within the complexity of the organization
   B. Day-to-day activities
   C. Looking to the future for the organization
   D. Personal accountability

8. Conceptual skills are essential for senior managers, including good judgment, intuition, creativity, problem-solving, coordinating various organizational functions, and _____.
   A. Accounting
   B. Inventory control
   C. Cost reporting
   D. Effective planning

9. Evidence shows that an individual can generally develop effective leadership capabilities by developing new habits to guide their behavior, learning the principles, skills, and techniques related to leadership, and translating those attributes and knowledge into _____.
   A. Changing the behaviors of others
   B. Meaningful activities and actions
   C. Direct customer service
   D. Achieving a deficiency-free survey

10. Jago's Leadership Research Matrix classifies leadership traits and behaviors, according to their organizational contexts, as either _____ or _____.
    A. Universal, situational
    B. Leadership, management
    C. Traditional, contemporary
    D. Internal, external

11. A health services executive's abilities, personality, and physical and social characteristics are considered leadership _____.
    A. Traits
    B. Qualities
    C. Behaviors
    D. Requirements

12. _____ research focuses on the conditions under which certain leadership traits are optimally effective.
    A. Characteristic
    B. Universal
    C. Situational
    D. Deontological

13. The _____ theory of leadership centers on two main assumptions: that leaders are born possessing certain traits that enable them to rise and lead and that the best leaders can arise when the need for them is highest.
    A. Transformational
    B. Great man
    C. Machiavellian
    D. Servant

14. Which of the following leadership models suggests that idealized influence, inspirational motivation, intellectual stimulation, and individualized consideration provide inspirational leadership for the organization?
    A. Leadership practices
    B. Leader exchange behavior
    C. Servant leadership
    D. Transformational leadership

15. According to transformational leadership theory, serving as a good role model concerning high ethical standards, instilling organizational pride, and earning high levels of respect is called _____.
    A. Intellectual stimulation
    B. Idealized influence
    C. Inspirational motivation
    D. Individualized consideration

16. A health services executive who uses group activities to facilitate people working together is engaging in _____ leadership.
    A. Participative
    B. Enlightened
    C. Facilitative
    D. Contemporary

17. An emotional intelligence (EI) quotient measures a person's capacity for awareness, control, and expression of one's emotions and for handling _____ judiciously and empathetically.
    A. Crisis situations
    B. Interpersonal relationships
    C. Stressful interactions
    D. Difficult conversations

18. Three fundamental leadership practices that correlate with a senior living organization's overall performance are communicating effectively, encouraging growth and innovation, and _____.
    A. Providing evidence supporting pay ranges
    B. Distributing sacrifices and rewards evenly
    C. Recognizing seniority
    D. Setting a clear vision for the future

19. Extensive research by the Gallup organization found that the most important difference between a great manager and a great leader is one of _____.
    A. Focus
    B. Talent
    C. Skills
    D. Training

20. Dana and Yukl proposed that the shift in management skills should be considered with ascending responsibilities in which of the following sequences?
    A. Technical, conceptual, relational
    B. Relational, technical, conceptual
    C. Technical, relational, conceptual
    D. Conceptual, technical, relational

21. According to the Association of Undergraduate Programs in Health Administration's definition, "The administrator must have a firm commitment to a philosophy of _____ to the patient/resident population. His or her primary professional role is as a _____ of an institutional or service environment, the ultimate purpose of which is quality patient care."
    A. Minimum standards, manager and leader
    B. Customer service, advocate and representative
    C. Care and service, shaper and designer
    D. Compassion, guardian and protector

22. _____ is/are typically more focused on the development of strategic goals, and _____ is generally more involved with the execution of tactics and operational actions.
    A. Governance, leadership
    B. Leadership, management
    C. Stockholders, management
    D. Management, leadership

23. Four strategic questions that leadership should address as part of a SWOT (strengths, weaknesses, opportunities, and threats) evaluation are as follows: (a) What is currently working, and how can it be improved? (b) What is not working and needs attention? (c) What is not working and should perhaps be discontinued? (d) What are we _____
    A. Not doing and should consider starting?
    B. Doing that is losing money?
    C. Not doing that our competition is doing?
    D. Going to do until the strategic plan is done?

24. Business writer and leadership analyst Jim Collins coined a term to describe an organization's process for developing its vision around becoming the very best in its class at a service or product, popularly known as the _____.
    A. Hedgehog concept
    B. Good to great method
    C. Skunkworks supposition
    D. Butterfly belief

25. When establishing and fostering a corporate culture of embracing change, _____ and _____ link teams of people and motivate coworkers to contribute their efforts during transitions.
    A. Trust, accountability
    B. Affirmation, honesty
    C. Trust, integrity
    D. Accountability, respect

26. In managing change, top-down trust involves a health services executive trusting the _____, judgment, and motivation of others to successfully adapt.
    A. Patience
    B. Competence
    C. Fortitude
    D. Loyalty

27. Fostering successful change is contingent on at least five factors: communication (open, frequent, and ongoing), proper training, stakeholder involvement in planning, consistency, and _____.
    A. Equal access to information
    B. Feedback channels
    C. Financial support
    D. Legal review

28. Action research suggests that there is an advantage gained when an organization embraces a formal approach for analyzing a situation, identifying possible solutions, and determining the best course of action based on the _____ to drive actions toward a solution.
    A. SWOT (strengths, weaknesses, opportunities, and threats) analysis
    B. Competitive environment
    C. Nature of the situation
    D. Current capacity

29. As part of the change process, the value of the timing—concerning when to share how much information with employees—cannot be _____.
    A. Predicted
    B. Expected
    C. Revealed
    D. Underestimated

30. The chief role of the health services executive in managing change is to _____, understanding that they will need to be a cheerleader during the initial phases of any change and responsible for sharing regular updates.
    A. Set strict expectations
    B. Establish disciplinary consequences for noncompliance
    C. Encourage an open and honest environment
    D. Provide incentives for adoption of the proposed change

31. When people understand and are excited about the direction of their organization, the likelihood of its operating margins rising above the median among its peers can actually _____.
    A. Double
    B. Decline
    C. Triple
    D. Stabilize

32. Innovative leadership includes both adopting _____ leadership and learning how to create an organizational climate where employees apply innovative thinking to solve problems and develop new products and services.
    A. A stable style of
    B. An innovative approach to
    C. Proven techniques for
    D. A core theory on

33. It is critically important to _____ the everyday efforts and successes of the management team and staff, as well as the organization's other critical stakeholders.
    A. Monitor
    B. Participate in
    C. Respect
    D. Celebrate

34. The marketing practice of creating a name, symbol, or design that identifies and differentiates a product or service from others is called _____.
    A. Expansion
    B. Penetration
    C. Public relations
    D. Branding

35. Increased competition and broadening consumer choices in the healthcare sector moved provider organizations toward adopting marketing strategies by the _____.
    A. 1930s
    B. Middle of the 20th century
    C. Turn of the 21st century
    D. Use of outside communications firms

36. Marketing is the process or technique of researching, promoting, _____, and distributing a product or service.
    A. Selling
    B. Packaging
    C. Pricing
    D. Presenting

37. _____ is one subset component of _____.
    A. Sales, promotion
    B. Promotion, marketing
    C. Marketing, promotion
    D. Marketing, public relations

38. Someone other than the consumer of a senior living service may _____ the decision to select a provider.
    A. Actually make
    B. Heavily influence
    C. Legally control
    D. All of the above

39. _____ is a strategic communication process that builds mutually beneficial relationships between an organization and multiple audiences.
    A. Marketing
    B. Public relations
    C. Promotion
    D. Branding

40. Which of the following is *not* an activity likely to be included in an organization's public relations strategy?
    A. Newsworthy press release
    B. Classified ad: employment sign-on bonus
    C. Social media post: quality award
    D. Personal interest story: resident/client

41. _____ encompasses the various methods and approaches an organization uses to establish and maintain a mutually beneficial relationship with the community in which it operates.
    A. Market segmentation
    B. Partnership stratification
    C. Community relations
    D. Community cultivation

42. Which of the following provides the most direct example of an organization's formal community relations program?
    A. Civic club membership
    B. Trade association leadership
    C. Little League team sponsorship
    D. Neighborhood watch participation

43. Market assessment and research are integrally linked to developing an organization's overarching _____.
    A. Strategic plan
    B. Marketing projections
    C. Public relations tactics
    D. Operating budget

44. A popular qualitative technique for conducting marketing research assembles between 6 and 12 individuals who might be existing customers, prospects, or decision-makers and provides a moderator to facilitate discussion about a product or service, referred to as a _____.
    A. Focus group
    B. Market test set
    C. Service development lab
    D. Delphi process group

45. _____ involves leveraging and utilizing the key information assets within an organization and aligning its mission and vision with its branding, messaging, and other visible marketing tools.
    A. Intramarket segmenting
    B. External marketing
    C. Internal audience cultivation
    D. Internal marketing

46. _____ focuses on keeping an organization's name visible in the community.
    A. Advertising
    B. Internal marketing
    C. Limelight promotion
    D. External marketing

47. The traditional marketing mix of the four Ps—product, price, promotion, and _____—applies to senior living with some unique and important twists.
    A. People
    B. Place
    C. Persistence
    D. Parity

48. The range and distribution of services offered by a senior living organization is known as its _____.
    A. Cafeteria plan
    B. Case mix
    C. Product mix
    D. Service span

49. _____ is creating a unique name and image for a product or service in a consumer's mind, mainly through advertising campaigns with a consistent theme and repetition.
    A. Marketing
    B. Branding
    C. Promoting
    D. Advertising

50. "Top-of-mind awareness" (TOMA) refers to a service or product brand being first in customers' minds when thinking of competing services or products; in the senior living arena, this is known as the _____ provider.
    A. Most remembered
    B. Best value
    C. Most trusted
    D. Highest quality

51. It is important to distinguish during the sales cycle the difference between a provider's _____, the menu and description of offered services, and _____, the relevance of each service to the prospective consumer.
    A. Prices, value
    B. Benefits, features
    C. Features, accessibility
    D. Features, benefits

52. An organization's marketing plan should be adequately resourced with time and money, be practical, focus on specific outcomes, and have both a method and a/an/the _____ to determine success.
    A. Deadline
    B. Means
    C. Metrics
    D. Advocate

53. Senior living marketing plans once emphasized giveaways or other special gift packages as tools to attract customers, but now that strategy is eroding in favor of a focus on building relationships with consumers and referral partners as well as using _____ to connect with potential customers.
    A. Advertising
    B. Technology
    C. Direct mail
    D. Social media

54. The health services executive must bolster the marketing knowledge and skills of the staff charged with planning and implementing the organization's marketing program by committing to _____.
    A. Hire additional staff
    B. Accountability for the marketing staff
    C. Support regular marketing training
    D. Technology investment

55. The responsibility of marketing ultimately rests with the _____ of a senior living provider organization.
    A. CEO/administrator
    B. Governing board
    C. Entire staff
    D. Licensed social worker

56. In the Deming PDCA performance improvement cycle, the step that involves gathering data about the change attempted is labeled _____.
    A. "P" for plan
    B. "A" for act
    C. "D" for do
    D. "C" for check

57. The "C" for "check" in the Deming PDCA cycle is sometimes expressed as an "S," which stands for _____.
    A. Scrutinize
    B. Study
    C. Synthesize
    D. Synchronize

58. Which of the following considerations would likely be the most compelling for someone to accept an invitation to serve on a problem-solving team?
    A. Whether there is more than one team forming to work on the problem.
    B. What might happen if the problem remains unaddressed?
    C. How the challenge relates to the organization's mission.
    D. Who benefits the most by solving the problem?

59. Communication involves a commitment of attention and time to both listening and _____ others through a variety of mediums, including personal conversations, meetings, and written commentary.
    A. Hearing
    B. Responding to
    C. Understanding
    D. Affirming

60. A health services executive must communicate effectively through a variety of information-sharing tools in order to bring the entire organization along with developing, implementing, and _____ changes and solutions.
    A. Defending
    B. Explaining
    C. Supporting
    D. Sustaining

61. Moving seamlessly between an organization's strategic initiatives and the daily demands of leading operations requires a health services executive to proactively develop and implement solutions that continuously improve the organization's performance, otherwise known as _____.
    A. Execution
    B. Total quality management
    C. Success
    D. Quality assurance and performance improvement

62. McChesney, Covey, and Huling concluded in their "4 Disciplines of Execution" that an effective leader identifies the most important goals, establishes lead measures for determining success, clearly assigns responsibility, and _____ on a regular basis.
    A. Communicates
    B. Keeps score
    C. Observes
    D. Receives reports

63. Together, accountability and _____ play important roles when monitoring the performance of the organization.
    A. Reward
    B. Incentives
    C. Attitude
    D. Alignment

64. The regular monitoring of an organization's business outcomes—service quality, human resources, and financial results—is known as _____.
    A. Output measurement
    B. Operational assessment
    C. Results review
    D. Metrics mirroring

65. Employee retention is considered a _____ measure of organizational performance.
    A. Lag
    B. Lead
    C. Contributing
    D. Causal

66. During the 1970s and 1980s, referred to as the senior living field's _____ era, providers responded to the growth in complexity of financing and regulatory systems by focusing more attention on operating efficiencies and standardization.
    A. Golden
    B. Business
    C. Big Bang
    D. Debutante

67. Business author Joseph Juran describes "_____" thinking as focusing narrowly on specific outcomes or tasks, such as clinical measures and survey deficiencies.
    A. Near horizon
    B. Big Q
    C. Little q
    D. Little e

68. _____ thinking, according to business author Joseph Juran, requires a broader view to develop systems that align all functions of the organization to contribute to performance excellence and customer satisfaction.
    A. Big Q
    B. Far horizon
    C. Little q
    D. Big E

69. Visionary thinking in senior living connects the best care and service practices to clients' _____, productivity to satisfied _____, and person-centered culture change to the rigor of managing effective processes and systems.
    A. Needs, clients
    B. Desires, owners
    C. Expectations, employees
    D. Expectations, regulators

70. The Baldrige Program is the nation's public–private partnership dedicated to recognizing organizational _____.
    A. Commitment to quality
    B. Strength and stability
    C. Consistency and performance
    D. Performance excellence

71. The primary aim of _____ is an increase in organizational performance by decreasing process variation.
    A. Lean management
    B. Six Sigma
    C. Black Belt Beta
    D. The process cycle

72. Lean management's core idea is to maximize customer value while minimizing _____.
    A. Down time
    B. Waste
    C. Cost
    D. Errors

73. Stephen Covey described four quadrants of time management with two planes: importance and _____.
    A. Urgency
    B. Difficulty
    C. Complexity
    D. Time investment

74. Regardless of service line, the National Association of Long Term Care Administrator Boards' (NAB's) core competencies are customer care, supports, and services; human resources; finance; environment; and _____.
    A. Person-centered care
    B. Information and technology
    C. Management and leadership
    D. Governance and leadership

75. Knowledge and skills concerning the systems that provide for a consistent, fair, and predictable method of job development and the recruitment, hiring, training, evaluating, and retaining of staff are essential for mastering the National Association of Long Term Care Administrator Boards' (NAB's) _____ domain.
    A. Talent acquisition and development
    B. Personnel management
    C. Person-centered leadership
    D. Human resources

76. Developing, implementing, and evaluating the senior living organization's contractual agreements, insurance, and risk management programs fits best in which of the following National Association of Long Term Care Administrator Boards (NAB) domains?
    A. Finance
    B. Environment
    C. Operations
    D. Management and leadership

77. Skills and knowledge about infection control and sanitation, emergency and disaster preparedness, and Health Insurance Portability and Accountability Act–compliant technology infrastructure are included in the National Association of Long Term Care Administrator Boards' (NAB's) domain known as _____.
    A. Operations
    B. Finance
    C. Environment
    D. Management and leadership

78. In addition to demonstrating knowledge and skills about ensuring compliance with applicable federal and state laws, rules, and regulations, the health services executive must meet the requirements of the National Association of Long Term Care Administrator Boards' (NAB's) _____ domain: developing, implementing, monitoring, and evaluating policies and procedures that reflect the organization's mission, values, and vision.
    A. Management and leadership
    B. Administration
    C. Customer care, supports, and services
    D. Quality assurance and performance improvement

79. Academic programs in long-term care administration are most commonly anchored in a higher education institution's college, school, or division of _____, health professions or public health, or arts and sciences.
    A. Nursing
    B. Social work
    C. Business
    D. Communications

80. Accreditation by the National Association of Long Term Care Administrator Boards of an academic program in long-term care administration requires an objective external assessment of an academic program's curriculum— including an experiential learning component (internship) of at least _____—faculty qualifications, staffing and other resources, institutional and provider community support, graduation rate, and student performance on the licensure exam.
    A. 1,000 hours
    B. Two semesters
    C. 400 hours
    D. One calendar year

81. Two nongovernmental organizations that offer support and guidelines for academic programs in health services administration are the Association of Undergraduate Programs in Health Administration (AUPHA) and _____.
    A. The Joint Commission
    B. The Commission on Accreditation for Healthcare Management Education (CAHME)
    C. The American College of Health Care Administrators
    D. The American Health Care Association

82. According to the National Association of Long Term Care Administrator Boards' (NAB's) professional practice analysis, over _____% of the knowledge and skills needed to effectively lead a senior living organization were the same across the continuum of postacute care.
    A. 55
    B. 82
    C. 90
    D. 76

83. In launching the health services executive initiative, the National Association of Long Term Care Administrator Boards (NAB) committed to addressing the challenges of bolstering the profession's image, minimizing inconsistent practice standards, meeting the needs of employers and regulators, supporting the NAB's member regulatory boards and agencies in their role of public protection, and _____.
    A. Creating a national continuing education standard
    B. Preventing licensure fraud and abuse
    C. Elevating licensure eligibility requirements
    D. Improving licensure portability

84. The National Association of Long Term Care Administrator Boards' health services executive (HSE™) qualification requires one to meet or exceed the education, experience, and examination requirements for licensure in most jurisdictions to practice as a nursing home administrator, as an assisted living administrator, or as an administrator of home- and community-based services; a state board that recognizes this credential for the purpose of issuing a professional license characterizes this approach as "licensure by _____."
    A. Reciprocity
    B. Endorsement
    C. Equivalency
    D. Reaffirmation

85. The professional society for executives who lead healthcare organizations, predominantly in acute care settings, known and respected in the field for its credentialing and educational programs, career development and public policy programs, and publishing division, the Health Administration Press, is called the _____.
    A. American College of Healthcare Executives (ACHE)
    B. American College of Health Care Administrators (ACHCA)
    C. Academy of Long Term Care Leadership and Development
    D. National Healthcare Managers Association

86. Human resources managers working in the senior living arena find great utility in developing a professional network through membership in the Society for Human Resources Management, the _____, or both.
    A. American Society for Health Care Human Resources Administration (ASHHRA)
    B. Healthcare Personnel Managers Association
    C. American College of Health Care Administrators (ACHCA)
    D. Society for Human Capital in Healthcare

87. A trade association differs from a professional society in that it represents the interests of _____, not those of individuals.
    A. Residents and their families
    B. Investors and governing boards
    C. Member organizations
    D. The communities served

88. Steven Covey suggested that the best investment a leader can make in their future is to develop and embrace a balanced program for self-renewal in the four areas of life: physical, social/emotional, mental, and _____.
    A. Financial
    B. Spiritual
    C. Relational
    D. Familial

ANSWERS AND RATIONALES

1. Answer: **C.** An organizational chart—showing reporting relationships and relative rank by position—is a derivative of the "specialized role" view of leadership; everyone has a job with specified responsibilities and related authority.

2. Answer: **A.** Formal titles do not always adequately reflect the functional dynamics of the group. Informal relationships and institutional history often play important roles in shaping who is viewed within the group as the leader for a given project or circumstance.

3. Answer: **D.** Advancing the organization's mission is a central tenet of leadership.

4. Answer: **A.** Processes applied for leadership versus management differ distinctively.

5. Answer: **B.** Providing a rationale for *why* a process exists is increasingly expected among today's workforce.

6. Answer: **C.** Management focuses on current operations meeting established performance goals.

7. Answer: **C.** Leadership envisions and articulates a brighter, compelling future for the organization.

8. Answer: **D.** Looking ahead and articulating a vision for the organization's future inspire others to engage in the successful pursuit of the mission.

9. Answer: **B.** Practical application is a true litmus test for developing leadership capabilities.

10. Answer: **A.** Answer is supported by the following: Jago, A. G. (1982). Leadership: Perspectives in theory and research. *Management Science, 28*(3), 315–337.

11. Answer: **A.** Traits are generally associated with naturally occurring characteristics—ones with which someone is born.

12. Answer: **C.** "Situational" derives its name from recognizing that circumstances—scale and context, history and evolving opportunities, and so forth—influence what leadership style or approach is most likely to be effective.

13. Answer: **B.** Historian Thomas Carlyle claimed that the world's story is a compilation of the biographies of great men.

14. Answer: **D.** These four elements form the basis of an inspirational leader's ability to "transform" an organization's culture.

15. Answer: **B.** Idealized influence is a foundational element of transformational leadership.

16. Answer: **A.** Enticing stakeholders to work together by practicing—and demonstrating that they are collectively contributing to the cause—attracts their continuing participation.

17. Answer: **B.** The ability to manage interpersonal relationships is a central component of the EI quotient.

18. Answer: **D.** People want and need to know the direction in which the organization is heading.

19. Answer: **A.** Focus on the big picture distinguishes a great leader.

20. Answer: **C.** Mastery first of the discipline or department (technical), then building proficiency in personal relationships (relational), and applying knowledge and skills in new ways (conceptual). Dana, B. (2005). *Developing a quality management system: The foundation for performance excellence in long term care.* AHCA; Yukl, G. (2006). *Leadership in organizations, 6e.* Prentice-Hall.

21. Answer: **C.** Answer is supported at the following website: www.aupha.org.

22. Answer: **B.** Leadership envisions and articulates a brighter, compelling future for the organization.

23. Answer: **A.** The first three questions are associated with strengths, weaknesses, and threats, respectively; this response is associated with opportunities.

24. Answer: **A.** Answer is supported in the following: Collins, J. (2001). *Good to great.* HarperCollins (pp. 90–119).

25. Answer: **C.** People value and are more likely to follow a leader they can trust and who has high integrity.

26. Answer: **B.** The leader must have confidence in the team members' abilities and professional competence in order to initiate and sustain meaningful change.

27. Answer: **B.** Evaluating progress requires some mechanism for gathering intelligence from end users and stakeholders affected by the change.

28. Answer: **C.** There is rarely a "one glove fits all hands," so complementing a standardized process with information that is truly unique to the situation is important.

29. Answer: **D.** Timing is perhaps as important as the content to be shared.

30. Answer: **C.** Anything less than an open and honest environment presents avoidable risks or low participation and/or buy-in by stakeholders.

31. Answer: **A.** Answer is supported in the following: Nautin, T. (2014). *The aligned organization.* McKinsey. www.mckinsey.com/business-functions/operations/our-insights/the-aligned-organization

32. Answer: **B.** An innovative approach to leadership contributes to the development of an organizational culture that values innovation.

33. Answer: **D.** Celebrating is an effective form of recognition and builds momentum.

34. Answer: **D.** An effective brand strategy provides the organization with a favorable edge in a competitive market.

35. Answer: **C.** Senior living options rose exponentially in the 70s and 80s and the accompanying rise in the number of potential customers triggered greater competition which led to a fuller adoption of marketing practices over the next couple of decades.

36. Answer: **A.** Marketing and sales are two business functions that are commonly tied closely together, even in naming the department responsible for them.

37. Answer: **B.** Marketing is the process or technique of researching, promoting, selling, and distributing a product or service.

38. Answer: **D.** Each of the scenarios is plausible and happens in senior living.

39. Answer: **B.** The term "public" relations implies external audiences.

40. Answer: **B.** A public relations strategy typically aims to elevate the organization's community image.

41. Answer: **C.** The community relations department builds and maintains positive and sustainable relationships in its communities with key individuals, groups, and organizations.

42. Answer: **C.** Sponsoring a team is both advertising and supporting a community-based activity with high visibility.

43. Answer: **A.** The strategic plan is the most "overarching" option listed.

44. Answer: **A.** Market research focus groups are controlled interviews of a target audience that are led by facilitators.

45. Answer: **D.** Marketing starts in one's own back yard—developing consistent messaging for ultimate use in the external marketing and sales efforts.

46. Answer: **D.** The keyword is "external."

47. Answer: **B.** The four Ps are considered (a) the product (the good or service); (b) the price (what the consumer pays); (c) promotion (advertising); and (d) the place (location where a product or service is provided or marketed).

48. Answer: **C.** Product mix, also known as product (or service) assortment, refers to the number of product or service lines a company offers to its customers and in what proportion to one another. The four dimensions to a company's product mix are width, length, depth, and consistency.

49. Answer: **B.** Marketing, promotion, and advertising activities can all contribute to building an organization's brand.

50. Answer: **A.** TOMA refers to thinking of the organization first—awareness (not necessarily qualitative ranking).

51. Answer: **D.** The most successful sales personnel typically focus on how the consumer will benefit from specific features offered by the organization.

52. Answer: **C.** It is essential to define "success" in order to know whether performance has met expectations.

53. Answer: **B.** Neither advertising nor direct mail builds relationships—they provide information; social media is one form of technology.

54. Answer: **C.** Continuous quality improvement is not limited to clinical roles—encouraging learning about new tools and techniques that can enhance performance in the marketing program is typically a wise investment.

55. Answer: **A.** The keyword is "ultimate"; authority can be delegated; responsibility rests with the leader.

56. Answer: **D.** During the Check phase, the data and results gathered from the Do phase are evaluated. Data are compared with the expected outcomes to see any similarities and differences.

57. Answer: **B.** While Deming marketed the quality improvement cycle he attributed to Shewhart, most people refer to it as the Deming cycle; the Study step involves measuring and analyzing the process or outcome of the Do step.

58. Answer: **C.** Contributing meaningfully to the overall success of the organization in pursuing its mission is the greatest draw of the four response options.

59. Answer: **B.** Communication requires a sender, a receiver, and feedback/verification.

60. Answer: **D.** Once implemented, sustaining a desired change is important in order to reap the benefits of the change.

61. Answer: **A.** The Medieval Latin root of "executive" is *exsequi*, which means "carry out," and so an executive carries out plans and actions.

62. Answer: **B.** Keeping track regularly of progress so that all stakeholders remain aware is key to succeeding. McChesney, C., Huling, J., & Covey, S. (2012). *The 4 disciplines of execution: Achieving your wildly important goals*. Free Press.

63. Answer: **D.** People who feel aligned with the organization's mission, values, and vision typically outperform those who feel less so.

64. Answer: **B.** Whether a full program review or an individual function review, stepping back to evaluate how a functional area or program is operating can provide invaluable insight for gaining efficiencies, identifying and prioritizing needed enhancements, and/or operating at a higher quality level.

65. Answer: **A.** Lag indicators are typically output oriented and easy to measure but challenging to improve or influence.

66. Answer: **B.** Senior living leaders began to see the need for an efficient and organized approach to respond to the growth in complexity of financing and regulatory systems.

67. Answer: **C.** Big Q requires broader thinking to develop systems that align all functions of the organization to contribute to performance excellence and customer satisfaction.

68. Answer: **A.** In contrast to big Q, little q thinking focuses narrowly on specific outcomes or tasks, such as clinical measures and survey deficiencies.

69. Answer: **C.** Clients' expectations should drive quality performance goals, and how well they are executed depends on the collective productivity of the staff team.

70. Answer: **D.** Answer is supported in the following: The Baldrige Performance Excellence Program, available at www.nist.gov/baldrige.

71. Answer: **B.** Six Sigma uses a methodology of define, measure, analyze, improve, and control.

72. Answer: **B.** Waste, or *muda* in Japanese, is defined as the performance of unnecessary work as a result of errors, poor organization, or communication.

73. Answer: **A.** The central message is to be proactive and spend as much time as possible on the important matters, especially those that are *both* important and urgent.

74. Answer: **C.** As of 2020, NAB maintains five core domains, one of which is "management and leadership."

75. Answer: **D.** The answer follows according to the NAB Candidate Handbook, available at www.nabweb.org/filebin/pdf/NAB_Handbook_October_2019 _WEB.pdf.

76. Answer: **A.** The answer follows according to the NAB Candidate Handbook, available at www.nabweb.org/filebin/pdf/NAB_Handbook_October_2019 _WEB.pdf.

77. Answer: **C.** The answer follows according to the NAB Candidate Handbook, available at www.nabweb.org/filebin/pdf/NAB_Handbook_October_2019 _WEB.pdf.

78. Answer: **A.** The answer follows according to the NAB Candidate Handbook, available at www.nabweb.org/filebin/pdf/NAB_Handbook_October_2019 _WEB.pdf.

79. Answer: **C.** Long-term care administration is about the "business" of senior living.

80. Answer: **A.** 1,000 hours is roughly the full-time equivalent of 6 months.

81. Answer: **B.** CAHME accredits graduate academic programs in health services administration, and AUPHA certifies undergraduate programs.

82. Answer: **B.** See Lindner, R. (2015). *NAB's professional practice analysis aligns leadership core competencies across expanding continuum of care* (White Paper). National Association of Long Term Care Administrator Boards.

83. Answer: **D.** Moving from one licensing jurisdiction to another became more and more complex due to the patchwork quilt of state laws and regulations governing licensure of administrators in senior living.

84. Answer: **C.** A state board that recognizes an applicant holding the HSE™ qualification accepts their knowledge, skills, and experience as "equivalent" to the standards it has established for issuing a license.

85. Answer: **A.** ACHE members work predominately in the acute care or hospital field; the remaining alternative response options relate to a professional society for long term care administrators (ACHCA) and its affiliated leadership program (Academy of Long Term Care Leadership and Development), or are fictitious (National Healthcare Managers Association).

86. Answer: **A.** Founded in 1964, the ASHHRA is a professional membership group of the American Hospital Association and has more than 2,500 members nationwide.

87. Answer: **C.** None of the alternate response options reflect organizations providing senior living services.

88. Answer: **B.** Expanding spiritual self through meditation, music, art, prayer, and/or service is the fourth area of self-renewal recommended by Covey.

PART II

Practice Exams

Provide Exams

CHAPTER 7

Core of Knowledge Practice Exam

1. An effective health services executive becomes knowledgeable (not necessarily an expert) about _____, the study of human aging.
   A. Gerontology
   B. Psychology
   C. Sociology
   D. Humanity

2. The ability of different computer platforms and programs to effectively use shared information is known as what?
   A. Shared services
   B. Proper channels
   C. Statistical Package for the Social Sciences (SPSS)
   D. Interoperability

3. The two main categories of interdisciplinary teams are _____ and _____ services.
   A. Clinical, technical
   B. Clinical, support
   C. Expert, support
   D. Expert, technical

4. The most prevalent aging-related conditions are diseases of the _____ system.
   A. Digestive
   B. Cardiovascular
   C. Nervous
   D. Respiratory

5. Exercising mental skills involving abstract reasoning, spatial relations, and perceptual speed is known as applying _____ intelligence.
   A. Fluid
   B. Acquired
   C. Crystallized
   D. Calculating

6. Mental skills that involve verbal memory and meaning, social judgment, and manipulating numbers are collectively known as known as _____ intelligence.
   A. Acquired
   B. Fluid
   C. Calculating
   D. Crystallized

7. The most prevalent mental disorder accompanying advanced age is _____.
   A. Dementia
   B. Anxiety
   C. Depression
   D. Delirium

8. The application of technology to health data collection, storage and retrieval, interpretation, and operational implementation is known as _____.
   A. Health information technology
   B. Artificial intelligence
   C. Personal health information
   D. Interoperability

9. HIPAA stands for _____.
   A. Health Insurance Portability and Accountability Act
   B. Health Information Protection and Accountability Act
   C. Health Insurance Preservation and Administration Act
   D. Healthcare Interdisciplinary Professions Agreement Act

10. The most widely recognized standards for measuring the degree of meaning-ful use achieved among two or more health information technology platforms are developed and maintained by the _____.
    A. World Health Organization
    B. American Health Information Management Association
    C. American National Standards Institute
    D. Health Level Seven International

11. The core goals of the Health Information Technology for Economic and Clinical Health Act were improving quality, safety, efficiency, and care coordination; ensuring adequate privacy for personal health information; and _____.
    A. Increasing the speed of information flow
    B. Assuring accountability
    C. Reducing health disparities
    D. Eliminating surprise billing

12. The level of academic preparation required currently to become a physical therapist is a _____ degree.
    A. Doctoral
    B. Master's
    C. Bachelor's
    D. Postdoctoral

13. The disorders most commonly reported to podiatrists by older adults are toe deformities, nail conditions, calluses, and _____.
    A. Fallen arches
    B. Fungal infections
    C. Neuropathy
    D. Corns

14. The most frequently diagnosed and treated vision conditions in older adults are macular degeneration, glaucoma, diabetic retinopathy, and _____.
    A. Cataracts
    B. Color blindness
    C. Shingles
    D. Histoplasmosis

15. The interdisciplinary study of the design, development, adoption, and application of information technology–based innovations in healthcare services delivery is known as _____.
    A. Artificial intelligence
    B. Health informatics
    C. Health information technology
    D. Electronic health record

16. When there is a reasonable probability of coming into contact with blood or other body fluids, nonintact skin, or mucous membranes, the Centers for Disease Control and Prevention recommends safety procedures designed to reduce the risk of transmitting potentially harmful microorganisms, which are known as _____.
    A. Universal precautions
    B. Body substance isolation procedures
    C. Standard precautions
    D. Contact precaution procedures

17. With the exception of short-term, postacute care for rehabilitation, _____ conditions tend to drive utilization of senior living lines of service.
    A. Severe
    B. Cognitive
    C. Medically complex
    D. Chronic

18. The overriding emphasis of senior living is postacute _____, in contrast with the acute care health system's primary objective of _____ a disease or repairing an injury.
    A. Services, treating
    B. Care, curing
    C. Transition, eliminating
    D. Living, preventing

19. The cultural expectation that a health professional has rank or advantage—is in charge—due to having greater knowledge, skills, and resources for effectively addressing the care recipient's needs is referred to as _____.
    A. A power differential
    B. Provider envy
    C. Professional privilege
    D. Caregiver concession

20. According to a Commonwealth Fund–backed study, just over _____ of skilled nursing care providers either have adopted or are in the process of implementing person-centered care approaches to their operations.
    A. Two thirds
    B. Three quarters
    C. 80%
    D. One half

21. One key characteristic that is common to both the Greatest Generation (born between 1901 and 1927) and the Silent Generation (born between 1928 and 1945) is _____, which may be why a medical model of service delivery has survived for as long as it has in senior living.
    A. Consumerism
    B. Appreciation for service
    C. Respect for authority
    D. Valuing scientific advancement

22. Many market experts anticipate that Baby Boomers (born between 1946 and 1964) will have much _____ consumer expectations than their predecessors. These individuals have observed service levels and approaches accepted by their parents and felt underwhelmed.
    A. Lower
    B. Higher
    C. Softer
    D. Broader

23. With 10,000 Baby Boomers turning 65 every day for the next several years, this is a demographic phenomenon that will surely make a mark on how senior living customer service is defined, delivered, and _____.
    A. Provided
    B. Evaluated
    C. Viewed
    D. Organized

24. Senior consumers typically want to receive care from personnel who are competent, respectful, friendly, and _____.
    A. Energetic
    B. Loud enough
    C. Polite
    D. Available

25. Senior consumers and their families value communication that is timely, transparent, and _____.
    A. Convenient
    B. Written
    C. Understandable
    D. Repeatable

26. Quality treatment includes preserving privacy and _____. The physical layout of the caregiving environment must provide appropriate privacy for the customer, and staff training should emphasize the importance of consistently following procedures that protect individual privacy.
    A. Confidentiality
    B. Comfort
    C. Security
    D. Hope

27. A health service executive should strive to develop and maintain an organizational culture that enables every customer to reasonably expect that information about their condition, treatment, prospects, or pay source is shared *only* with persons who are directly involved with their care, work for a government agency with regulatory oversight authority, or are _____.
    A. Related by blood
    B. Insurance company employees
    C. Authorized by the customer to have access
    D. Related by marriage

28. Basic human comforts typically include shelter, nutrition and water, and community, such as social engagement opportunities that _____.
    A. Maximize a person's prospects for functional independence
    B. Foster an attitude of optimism and hope
    C. Enhance the healing process
    D. Minimize the risk of isolation, loneliness, or boredom

29. Coined by MyInnerView, Inc., as the "_____ Question," it is considered the single most useful gauge on the provider's customer dashboard: "How likely are you to recommend this provider to someone you know who is searching for the same services?"
    A. Bottom Line
    B. Enlightened
    C. Ultimate
    D. Litmus Test

30. What distinguishes contemporary health services executives among their peers is the extent to which they constantly exercise imagination to _____ core values in fresh ways that help embed them in the mind-set of everyone on the team.
    A. Validate
    B. Demonstrate
    C. Reveal
    D. Strengthen

31. A Medicare- and Medicaid-certified provider is not permitted by the Centers for Medicare & Medicaid Services to hire someone who _____.
    A. Is a convicted felon
    B. Has no government-issued photo ID
    C. Cannot speak English
    D. Needs special accommodation to perform the job

32. Key elements of a job offer include position title, work shift and location, starting date, compensation, and _____.
    A. An acceptance line for the candidate to sign and return
    B. Perks
    C. Opportunities for advancement
    D. A list of observed holidays

33. The federal form a new employee is required to complete to establish the appropriate level of tax withholdings is known as the _____ form.
    A. W-2
    B. IRS-2067
    C. I-9
    D. W-4

34. The federal form a new employee is required to complete in order to establish citizenship and employment eligibility is called the _____ form.
    A. W-4
    B. W-2
    C. I-9
    D. Schedule A

35. When staff members collaborate to set the work schedule among themselves, without a master scheduler, they form what is known as a _____.
    A. Bargaining unit
    B. Innovation cell group
    C. Self-directed work team
    D. Skunkworks squad

36. An effective position description conveys performance expectations that are clearly written and stipulates the essential duties of the position, reporting relationships, work site location, and _____.
    A. Time record procedure
    B. Physical demands
    C. Paid time-off policy
    D. Preemployment requirements

37. The Family Medical Leave Act allows an eligible employee to take _____ leave for a serious health condition of either the employee or an immediate family member for up to _____ weeks during a 12-month period.
    A. Paid, 6
    B. Unpaid, 9
    C. Paid, 12
    D. Unpaid, 12

38. Two key determinants of whether a benefit can be considered de minimis are its _____ and value.
    A. Frequency
    B. Transferability
    C. Availability
    D. Duration

39. The Fair Labor Standards Act classifies an employee whose primary duties focus on managing the enterprise or one of its departments and customarily and regularly directing the work of at least two employees and who has the authority to hire, fire, or change the status of other employees as _____.
    A. Exempt
    B. Professional
    C. Nonexempt
    D. Excluded

40. Human resources management includes assisting departments with recruiting, screening, hiring, orienting and onboarding, training, supporting, and _____ competent, motivated staff members.
    A. Paying
    B. Retaining
    C. Evaluating
    D. Scheduling

41. In order to receive a professional credential in the healthcare field, it is standard practice to require at least some demonstration of a person's command of the fundamental _____ essential to practicing a specific discipline.
    A. History and context
    B. Regulations and expectations
    C. Knowledge and skills
    D. Demand and prospects

42. Health professionals who must acquire a state-issued license to practice are typically expected to also engage in relevant _____ activities in order to periodically renew their license.
    A. Professional society
    B. Pro bono
    C. Preceptorship
    D. Continuing education

43. Attendance has at least two key characteristics: presence and _____.
    A. Engagement
    B. Punctuality
    C. Productivity
    D. Wellness

44. On any given day, a senior living organization with 100 employees could expect to have _____ staff members missing.
    A. 8
    B. 10
    C. 6
    D. 2

45. Recruiting, screening, _____, onboarding, compliance, training, and developing talent are fundamental functions of managing human resources.
    A. Hiring
    B. Terminating
    C. Paying
    D. Disciplining

46. The financial report that reflects an organization's business activity—revenues and expenses—over a period of time is called its _____.
    A. Balance sheet
    B. Cash flow statement
    C. Operating budget
    D. Income statement

47. The _____ is the internal financial document that illustrates an organization's fiscal health—a profile of its assets and liabilities at a point in time.
    A. Income statement
    B. Operating budget
    C. Balance sheet
    D. Audit report

48. How much money is needed to meet expenses and when as well as how much revenue will be collected and how fast is tracked and reported as an organization's _____.
    A. Capital budget
    B. Profit and loss statement
    C. Operating pro forma
    D. Cash flow statement

49. Which of the following measures is considered a profitability or margin ratio?
    A. Net operating ratio
    B. Debt service coverage
    C. Current ratio
    D. Capital spending ratio

50. An organization's ability to meet its annual debt services obligations is measured by its _____.
    A. Days cash on hand
    B. Debt-to-capitalization ratio
    C. Debt service coverage
    D. Accounts receivable

51. An operating budget includes both fixed and _____ expenses.
    A. Flexible
    B. Time-limited
    C. Variable
    D. Unanticipated

52. Which of the following items would not likely appear in a capital budget?
    A. Truckloads of adult briefs
    B. Commercial stove
    C. Rooftop chiller
    D. Telephone system

53. The capital structure for senior care and service properties comes from a few primary sources: debt, equity, lease capital, government programs, and _____.
    A. Community Development Block Grants
    B. Commercial lenders
    C. Industrial revenue bonds
    D. Donations

54. A Medicare Part C insurance policy is also called a Medicare _____ plan.
    A. Supplement
    B. Advantage
    C. Complement
    D. Rider

55. The section of the Medicare program that covers inpatient hospital care, limited postacute skilled nursing care (institutional or home health), and hospice services is known as Part _____.
    A. A
    B. B
    C. C
    D. D

56. Part __ of the Medicare program provides coverage for beneficiaries for medically necessary outpatient services that diagnose or treat a medical condition, preventive health services that detect or prevent illness, ambulance services, medical equipment, and some mental healthcare services.
    A. B
    B. A
    C. C
    D. D

57. Providing insurance to pay for enrolling in prescription drug plans is the purpose of Medicare Part _____.
    A. D
    B. B
    C. C
    D. A

58. The chief barriers to more people buying commercial long-term care insurance are skepticism about whether someone will ever need to file a claim, a generally unfavorable view of long-term care service options, an overstated expectation of the safety net provided by Medicare and Medicaid, and the perceived _____.
    A. Limited number of carriers
    B. Lack of access to quality providers
    C. High cost of premiums
    D. Difficulty of receiving benefits

59. A risk management element concerned with the electronic use, management, and transfer of patient and employee information is known as _____.
    A. Cybersecurity
    B. Informatics
    C. Artificial intelligence
    D. A firewall

60. An independent and objective analysis of an organization's financial reports to ensure that they accurately reflect its actual performance is called _____.
    A. An audit
    B. Its annual report
    C. The social impact statement
    D. Financial performance verification

61. The most widely accepted authority on standards for buildings—commercial or residential—to minimize the risk of harm to anyone who enters is the _____.
    A. Agency for Safety and Emergency Preparedness
    B. National Council on Building Codes and Standards
    C. American Institute of Architects
    D. National Fire Protection Association

62. The National Fire Protection Association-101 (NFPA-101) covers life safety in _____ structures.
    A. New and existing
    B. New
    C. Existing
    D. Occupied

63. A preventive maintenance program commonly includes systematic inspection, detection of irregularities or signs of wear and tear, and correction of identified problems, all with the common goal of _____.
    A. Avoiding expensive repairs
    B. Reducing the risk of failures
    C. Extending the useful life of capital assets
    D. Lowering workers' compensation claims

64. Electronically maintaining parallel sets of the same data—concerning patient care, personnel records, or business files—is referred to as _____.
    A. Redundancy
    B. Reinforcement
    C. Cut-and-paste
    D. Duplication

65. A hazard vulnerability analysis determines which hazards are the most likely to present a risk, the potential impact on the organization's operation at varying levels of severity, and its _____.
    A. Speed of corrective action
    B. Community support network
    C. Capacity for mounting an effective response
    D. Vehicular capacity for relocating residents

66. Which of the following hazard risks is not associated with a particular location or region for the purpose of developing hazard vulnerability analysis?
    A. Earthquake
    B. Wildfire
    C. Active aggressor
    D. Industrial accident

67. An effective price analysis process includes developing product specifications that objectively address quality grade, composition, availability, weight, and

    _____.
    A. Packaging
    B. Price
    C. Distribution
    D. Size

68. The section of the IRS code that permits donors to deduct contributions to the organization from their taxable income on their individual income tax returns is _____.
    A. 503(c)(1)
    B. C.501.3
    C. 501(c)(3)
    D. 501(3)(c)

69. _____ is a professional credential awarded by a governmental agency to recognize someone who meets minimal practice standards, and _____ is a professional credential awarded by a nongovernmental organization in recognition of demonstrating advanced professional knowledge and skills.
    A. Certification, licensure
    B. Licensure, certification
    C. Licensure, accreditation
    D. Accreditation, licensure

70. Disputes between individuals, between organizations, or between individuals and organizations fall into the legal category of _____ actions.
    A. Civil
    B. Criminal
    C. Tort
    D. Liability

71. A senior living leader should balance the organization's focus on marketing and customer service with the need to develop and institutionalize effective quality management systems that consistently _____ the expectations of the customers.
    A. Define and refine
    B. Support or refute
    C. Meet or exceed
    D. Validate and verify

72. _____ processes seek to produce predictability and order while _____ processes aim to produce organizational change.
    A. Management, leadership
    B. Supervisory, self-directed team
    C. Leadership, management
    D. Traditional, contemporary

73. Management is focused on _____, and leadership is focused on _____, both critically necessary for the survival of the organization.
    A. The macro, the micro
    B. Tomorrow, today
    C. Today, tomorrow
    D. Finances, quality

74. Leadership _____ are generally associated with characteristics with which you are born, such as personality or motivations, but _____ are more commonly tied to skills you have learned.
    A. Traits, behaviors
    B. Inherencies, proficiencies
    C. Behaviors, traits
    D. Aptitudes, talents

75. The four key assumptions of transformational leadership theory are intellectual stimulation, inspirational motivation, idealized influence, and _____.
    A. Individualized consideration
    B. Integrity optimization
    C. Insightful mentoring
    D. Integrated communication

76. The four key components of Goleman's emotional intelligence model are self-awareness, self-regulation, social awareness or skills, and _____.
    A. Executive judgment
    B. Emotional stability
    C. Technical proficiency
    D. Relationship management

77. Greenleaf's servant leadership model emphasizes the critical importance of a leader's vision and foresight, persuasiveness and commitment to people's growth, listening and communication skills, stewardship, and _____.
    A. Dedication to compliance
    B. Visible presence
    C. Intestinal fortitude
    D. Transparency

78. The Multifactor Leadership Questionnaire measures leadership practices that stimulate strong follower commitment, including the influence leaders have on followers' perception of problems, how leaders encourage and support followers, effectively communicate an appealing vision, model desired behaviors, and _____.
    A. Achieve fair and equal treatment
    B. Justify exceptions
    C. Enforce rules to avoid mistakes
    D. Monitor performance improvement

79. The Leadership Practices Inventory assesses how effectively a leader challenges current processes, empowers others to act, models the way forward, encourages people, and _____.
    A. Champions a shared vision
    B. Reduces waste and inefficiency
    C. Improves staff retention
    D. Strengthens social impact

80. An organization's _____ statement articulates the underlying principles it embraces.
    A. Mission
    B. Vision
    C. Social impact
    D. Values

81. The term "SWOT analysis" refers to assessing an organization's _____.
    A. Stresses, workforce, outcomes, and tactics
    B. Strategies, wherewithal, outcomes, and tactics
    C. Strengths, weaknesses, opportunities, and threats
    D. Stakeholders, weaknesses, opportunities, and threats

82. The Plan–Do–Check–Act model provides a disciplined _____ framework for developing an organization's strategic plan.
   A. And bidirectional
   B. Improvement cycle
   C. Three-dimensional
   D. And fluid

83. Stephen Covey suggested developing a clear vision of the organization's desired direction and destination by _____.
   A. Insisting on consensus within the leadership team
   B. Involving only key stakeholders
   C. Respecting resource limits
   D. Beginning with the end in mind

84. A popular goal-setting template that provides a simple, straightforward guide to help leaders successfully develop, initiate, and implement goals produces what are known as SMART goals, which stands for _____.
   A. Specific, measurable, assignable, realistic, and time-based
   B. Statistical metrics and reachable tasks
   C. Social measures for accountability and retrospective testing
   D. Specific, major, aspirational, reachable, and timely

85. To sustain high operational performance—clinical, financial, and regulatory compliance—it is important to understand and reduce _____ as much as possible.
   A. Costs
   B. Turnover
   C. Variation
   D. Inefficiency

86. As it relates to change management, bottom–up trust is based on the staff's perceptions of the health services executive's _____ and ability to perform well.
   A. Energy
   B. Patience
   C. Experience
   D. Integrity

87. The third step in Lewin's three-step model of organizational change, in which stabilization of the change occurs, is known as _____.
   A. Freezing
   B. Thawing
   C. Moving
   D. Refreezing

88. Lippett's model of organizational change underscores the _____ nature of change.
    A. Cyclical
    B. Linear
    C. Bidirectional
    D. Inevitable

89. What does TOMA stand for?
    A. Top-of-mind awareness
    B. Together our minds awaken
    C. Top of mental ability
    D. To offer marketing applications

90. Which is not one of the four Ps associated with marketing?
    A. Product
    B. People
    C. Price
    D. Promotion

91. _____ is comparing an organization's strengths and weaknesses to competitors' performance in the same service lines.
    A. Secret shopping
    B. Service mapping
    C. Benchmarking
    D. Market segmentation

92. The ability of a health services executive to make sound decisions by engaging in reflective and independent root cause analysis is referred to as _____.
    A. Algorithm assessment
    B. Critical thinking
    C. Delphi testing
    D. Soundness scrutiny

93. What do the letters "C" and "I" stand for in the six-step DECIDE performance improvement model?
    A. Consider (all alternatives) and identify (the best one)
    B. Clarify (options) and identify (the most likely to succeed)
    C. Create (a matrix of possibilities) and imagine (the best outcome)
    D. Consider (the cost of the status quo) and investigate (the benefits of change)

94. A problem-solving approach that uses cause-and-effect brainstorming to identify possible causes of a problem by sorting ideas into useful areas or categories produces as an illustrative work product a _____.
    A. Fishbone diagram
    B. Brainstorm form
    C. Delphi diagram
    D. Alpha algorithm

95. A contemporary management information tool that displays key performance indicators, metrics, and data points to facilitate monitoring the operational health of an organization is commonly referred to as a leadership _____.
    A. Barometer
    B. Compass
    C. Periscope
    D. Dashboard

96. The Baldrige model measures the degree to which an organization's leadership successfully applies its core values and management approach to integrating _____, customers, operations, and workforce.
    A. Tactics
    B. Strategy
    C. Goals
    D. Objectives

97. Six Sigma uses a methodology of define, measure, analyze, _____, and control.
    A. Improve
    B. Study
    C. Modify
    D. Verify

98. When a state licensure board accepts the National Association of Long Term Care Administrator Boards' (NAB's) health services executive qualification as fulfilling its licensure requirements for any postacute service line, it awards licensure by _____.
    A. Endorsement
    B. Reciprocity
    C. Equivalency
    D. Eminent privilege

99. The _____ is the professional society that specifically represents the interests of long-term care administrators throughout North America, providing educational programming, advocacy, and career development opportunities for its members.
    A. Academy of Long-Term Care Leadership
    B. American College of Healthcare Executives
    C. Society for Post-Acute and Long-Term Care Medicine
    D. American College of Health Care Administrators

100. Strategically planning one's continuing education journey with an eye toward enhancing existing skills and expertise, as well as building new ones, is called a _____.
    A. Professional development plan
    B. Career matrix
    C. Self-improvement map
    D. Career ladder

CHAPTER 8

Nursing Home Administration Practice Exam

1. When it comes to dining services, professional input from a _____ is required by Medicare, Medicaid, and many commercial insurers.
   A. Dietary manager
   B. Registered dietitian
   C. Head chef
   D. Culinary expert

2. The current name for the professional association representing the interests of long-term care medical directors is the _____.
   A. Society for Post-Acute and Long-Term Care Medicine
   B. American Physicians Practice
   C. America's Long-Term Care Physicians
   D. Society of Medical Directors

3. QAPI sets the stage for senior living providers to engage in an ongoing, organized method of conducting business to achieve optimum results. What does it stand for?
   A. Quality aspects of people investment
   B. Quality aptitude and progress improvement
   C. Quality assurance and performance improvement
   D. Quick assurance and progress investment

4. The Centers for Medicare & Medicaid Services and the Office of the National Coordinator for Health Information Technology describe the effective electronic exchange of health information as _____ use of the data.
   A. Practical
   B. Meaningful
   C. Pragmatic
   D. Beneficial

5. The two main categories of interdisciplinary teams in a skilled nursing facility setting are _____ services and _____ services.
   A. Multidisciplinary, clinical
   B. Clinical, support
   C. Transdisciplinary, support
   D. Person-centered, required

6. The medical professional who directly manages the care of a person in a skilled nursing facility is called their _____.
   A. Medical director
   B. Medical consultant
   C. Main doctor
   D. Attending physician

7. Senior living providers with service lines that participate in Medicare or Medicaid are expected by the Centers for Medicare & Medicaid Services to contract with a licensed _____ to serve as medical director.
   A. Nurse practitioner
   B. MD
   C. DO
   D. Physician

8. To become a certified nurse aide, one must pass a written exam and demonstrate satisfactory proficiency in providing personal care (such as oral care, bathing, and personal hygiene), performing several related tasks (such as proper body mechanics for lifting and transferring, handwashing, and making an occupied bed), and _____.
   A. Documenting a person's condition
   B. Measuring a person's vital signs
   C. Utilizing the electronic medical record
   D. Observing behavioral changes

9. The two most widely recognized credentials for a medical records technician working in a skilled nursing facility are Registered Health Information Technician and _____.
   A. Licensed Medical Records Technician
   B. Certified Professional Coder
   C. Registered Health Records Specialist
   D. Qualified Health Information Manager

10. According to the Centers for Medicare & Medicaid Services, a social worker for a Medicare-certified skilled nursing facility with more than 120 beds must hold at least a _____ degree in _____.
    A. Graduate, social work
    B. Associate, social sciences
    C. Bachelor's, social sciences
    D. Bachelor's, social work

11. The current name for the professional association formerly known as the American Medical Directors Association is the _____.
    A. International Medical Directors Association
    B. Physicians for ElderCare
    C. American Geriatricians Society
    D. Society for Post-Acute and Long-Term Care Medicine

12. The credential that requires a physician to demonstrate knowledge and skills regarding geriatric medicine and relevant regulatory compliance in long-term care settings is _____.
    A. Board-certified geriatrician
    B. Certified medical director
    C. Qualified postacute care physician
    D. Advanced geriatric practitioner

13. The development of the elements of the QAPI programs was largely supported by the _____.
    A. Health Service Research
    B. Centers for Disease Control and Prevention
    C. Centers for Medicare & Medicaid Services
    D. Department of Health and Human Services

14. QAPI programs typically target issues concerning comfort, safety, quality, and _____.
    A. Regulatory compliance
    B. Infection control
    C. Disaster preparedness
    D. Life satisfaction

15. An _____ assessment form is completed for each care recipient, regardless of payment source, upon admission and then periodically.
    A. Individual Service Plan
    B. Minimum Data Set
    C. Outcome and Assessment Information Set
    D. Patient Assessment Instrument

16. Each of the following describes a section of the Minimum Data Set except _____.
    A. Cardiovascular system
    B. Functional status
    C. Mood
    D. Restraints

17. The patient assessment tool used in a Medicare-certified inpatient rehabilitation facility is known as the _____.
    A. Minimum data set
    B. Patient Assessment Instrument
    C. Outcome and Assessment Information Set
    D. Individual Service Plan

18. The resident assessment tool used in a Medicare-certified skilled nursing facility is called the _____.
    A. Outcome and Assessment Information Set
    B. Individual Service Plan
    C. Minimum Data Set
    D. Patient Assessment Instrument

19. The Centers for Medicare & Medicaid Services (CMS) expects a provider's quality assurance and performance improvement program to include at least the following five elements: design and scope, governance and leadership, performance improvement projects, systematic analysis and systemic action, and _____.
    A. Feedback, data systems, and monitoring
    B. Emergency preparedness planning
    C. Corporate compliance and accountability
    D. Risk management, documentation, and privacy protection

20. The Centers for Medicare & Medicaid Services' (CMS's) Five-Star Quality Rating System for skilled nursing facilities includes three major components: compliance record, quality measures, and _____.
    A. Process metrics
    B. Staffing
    C. Consumer survey
    D. Clinical outcomes

21. A high-performing senior living organization establishes policies and procedures that enable it to receive real-time feedback from those it serves on every aspect of the operation that touched them—_____ or _____—as an essential element of its quality assurance and performance improvement program.
    A. During, afterward
    B. Clinically, financially
    C. Positively, negatively
    D. Large, small

22. Annual employee turnover in America's skilled nursing facilities has been estimated to be as high as _____.
    A. 100%
    B. 120%
    C. 55%
    D. 75%

23. The Institute of Medicine considers the optimal licensed nursing staff threshold for a skilled nursing facility caring for short-stay residents to be _____ hours per resident per day.
    A. 2.00
    B. 1.15
    C. 1.30
    D. 0.55

24. The Institute of Medicine considers the optimal threshold for nurse aide staff in a skilled nursing facility caring for long-stay residents to be _____ hours per resident per day.
    A. 2.00
    B. 1.15
    C. 0.75
    D. 2.80

25. The Centers for Medicare & Medicaid Services requires a Medicare/Medicaid-certified skilled nursing facility to have sufficient nursing staff to provide nursing and related services to attain or maintain the _____ physical, mental, and psychosocial well-being of each resident, as determined by resident assessments and plans of care.
    A. Most optimal
    B. Highest practicable
    C. Maximum attainable
    D. Most consistent

26. The Centers for Medicare & Medicaid Services requires Medicare- and Medicaid-certified long-term care providers to electronically submit direct care staffing information, called a _____.
    A. Self-Directed Schedule
    B. Direct Care Staffing Plan
    C. Schedule-Based Record
    D. Payroll-Based Journal

27. Effective from 1971, the federal government _____ that each state create a board of licensure for nursing home administrators.
    A. Mandated
    B. Recommended
    C. Requested
    D. Pursued

28. _____ is the federal–state healthcare financing program designed to support medically indigent Americans.
    A. Medicare
    B. Supplemental Security Income
    C. Medicaid
    D. Old Age Assistance

29. Someone who qualifies for participation in both Medicare and Medicaid is referred to as _____.
    A. Medically indigent
    B. Dually eligible
    C. Duel-eligible
    D. MM-qualified

30. A typical skilled nursing facility receives approximately one half of its revenue from _____.
    A. Medicare A and B
    B. Commercial health and long-term care insurance
    C. Privately paying consumers
    D. Medicaid

31. Some states require that the private pay rate for skilled nursing facility services cannot be greater than the daily Medicaid reimbursement; this is a public policy approach known as _____.
    A. Rate equalization
    B. Lower cost or charges
    C. Fairness doctrine
    D. Rate optimization

32. The two primary elements of the Medicare Patient-Driven Payment Model for skilled nursing facilities are the base rate and _____.
    A. Resource utilization group
    B. Case mix index
    C. Diagnosis-related group
    D. Minimum Data Set

33. Medicare's Patient-Driven Payment Model determines reimbursement rates based on a resident's _____ rather than the amount of care or services provided.
    A. Primary and secondary diagnosis
    B. Medical history and risks
    C. Condition and care needs
    D. Preferences and perceived needs

34. The Life Safety Code (National Fire Protection Association-101 [NFPA-101]) is either referenced or incorporated into federal, state, and local regulations governing construction, healthcare facility licensing, and _____.
    A. The approval of mortgage insurance offered by federal agencies
    B. The issuance of industrial revenue bonds
    C. Occupational safety and health
    D. Certification for participation in Medicare or Medicaid

35. Medical records of older adults are to be retained for at least _____.
    A. 5 years
    B. 6 years
    C. 3 years
    D. 10 years

36. The Life Safety Code (National Fire Protection Association-101 [NFPA-101]) requires a skilled nursing facility to have a sprinkler system and at least _____ areas that are separated by special fire-resistant building materials and fire-rated doors.
    A. Three
    B. Four
    C. Two
    D. Two or three

37. One of the most consistently cited regulatory violations among licensed postacute care communities is incomplete _____.
    A. Labels on food containers
    B. Disaster preparedness plans
    C. Medicaid recertification forms
    D. Health Insurance Portability and Accountability Act compliance records

38. Internal reports that a governing board should expect to regularly receive from a health services executive would address progress on meeting the goals stated in the strategic plan, quality assurance and performance improvement efforts, financial performance, regulatory compliance, risk management, client satisfaction, and _____.
    A. Medicaid rate adjustments
    B. Employee engagement
    C. Current and anticipated competition
    D. Unemployment statistics

39. The Centers for Medicare & Medicaid Services (CMS) publishes a set of Interpretive Guidelines for inspectors and skilled nursing facility providers to understand what is expected—how compliance with relevant regulations is determined—and which is more formally referred to as the _____.
    A. Watermelon Book
    B. Compliance Road Map
    C. CMS Health Insurance Manual (HIM)-15
    D. State Operations Manual

40. Which of the following headings is *not* included in the Centers for Medicare & Medicaid Services' Interpretive Guidelines?
    A. Resident Rights
    B. Comprehensive Person-Centered Care Plans
    C. Quality of Care
    D. Life Satisfaction

41. A Centers for Medicare & Medicaid Services (CMS) compliance survey of a skilled nursing facility can be performed periodically (typically 12–18 months apart) or in response to a _____.
    A. Natural disaster
    B. Complaint filed by a resident, family, or employee
    C. Negative newspaper report
    D. Lender inquiry

42. Surveys for state licensure and Medicare/Medicaid certification, recertification, and complaint investigations occur _____, and accreditation inspections typically take place _____.
    A. Without notice, by appointment
    B. Without notice, without notice
    C. By appointment, without notice
    D. Annually, by appointment

43. A key criticism of the enforcement approach employed by the Centers for Medicare & Medicaid Services is that little evidence exists to support its underlying assumption that _____.
    A. Timely revisits ensure compliance
    B. Penalties effectively deter poor-quality care
    C. A deficiency-free survey causes performance improvement
    D. B and C

44. A nursing home administrator is licensed as a health professional in every state and Washington, DC, due to a federal mandate that was included in amendments made to the _____.
    A. Older Americans Act
    B. Social Security Act
    C. Americans with Disabilities Act
    D. Health Professions Licensure Act

45. Under the federal mandate for each state to establish a licensure board for nursing home administrators, each board is required to develop and enforce standards that licensees are at least _____, otherwise suitable, and qualified to serve because of training or expertise in institutional administration.
    A. 21 years old
    B. Of good moral character
    C. A college graduate
    D. Free from any communicable disease

46. The impetus for forming the National Association of Long Term Care Administrator Boards in 1971 was the need for nursing home administrator licensure boards to _____.
    A. Share information and best practices
    B. Lobby state legislatures and Congress
    C. Develop a national qualifying examination
    D. Comply with federal regulations uniformly

47. Regardless of the formal education pathway, most licensing jurisdictions expect an applicant to complete a field learning tenureship prior to taking the licensure exam, which is often referred to as a/an _____ requirement.
    A. Administrative Fellowship
    B. Administrator-in-Training
    C. Leadership Apprenticeship
    D. Administrator Externship

48. The host organization's leader who serves as the experienced supervisor during an Administrator-in-Training practicum is most commonly called their _____.
    A. Field supervisor
    B. Adviser
    C. Guide
    D. Preceptor

49. Bidirectional acceptance of licensed nursing home administrators—one board accepting a licensee from another state's board if the recognition is mutual—is known as _____.
    A. Interstate consent
    B. Endorsement
    C. Reciprocity
    D. Professional compact

50. _____ occurs when a licensure board reviews an application submitted by a person who holds a license in good standing from another jurisdiction's board and determines that they meet all the expected requirements for a license—and the board waives any additional demonstration of skills or knowledge to issue a license.
    A. Interstate mobility
    B. Endorsement
    C. Reciprocity
    D. Deemed status.

CHAPTER 9

Residential Care and Assisted Living Practice Exam

1. What are the two different ways technology is used with the senior care field?
   A. Applied and nonapplied
   B. Applied and health information
   C. Basic and health information
   D. Basic and advanced

2. _____ now serves as a tremendous resource portal for any residential care and assisted living organization or person interested in learning more about culture change and person-centered and person-directed care, including training materials, current research, and high impact practices.
   A. The Voice of Change
   B. The Pioneer Way
   C. The Pioneer Network
   D. The Platform for Change

3. What is the fourth stage of culture change that the Commonwealth Fund identified through its research focused on the key elements in congregate living settings?
   A. Household
   B. Institutional
   C. Neighborhood
   D. Transformational

4. The top four leading causes of death among older Americans are heart disease, cancer, chronic obstructive pulmonary disease, and _____.
   A. Dementia
   B. Stroke
   C. Osteoporosis
   D. Suicide

5. Positive aging is characterized by preserving one's cognitive level, remaining socially engaged, coping with life's events, and _____.
   A. Renewing creative interests
   B. Achieving contentment
   C. Avoiding disability and disease
   D. Having sufficient financial resources

6. The importance of _____ wellness tends to increase with advancing age.
   A. Spiritual
   B. Financial
   C. Family
   D. Emotional

7. Titles such as Life Enrichment Director, Social Engagement Coordinator, and Life Quality Assistant are emerging replacements for the more traditional title of _____.
   A. Chaplain
   B. Resident Services Representative
   C. Activities Director
   D. Social Worker

8. One of the top challenges of providing routine dental treatment for residents of residential care and assisted living communities is _____.
   A. Access to transportation
   B. Low Medicaid reimbursement
   C. Poor oral hygiene habits
   D. Proximity to a dental office

9. The most valuable information a hair care professional working in a residential care or assisted living setting can provide to the interdisciplinary team concerns observed changes in a client's condition, capacity, or _____.
   A. Resources
   B. Balance
   C. Hearing
   D. Behavior

10. The interdisciplinary team has as its core purpose developing a comprehensive plan of care with clearly stated and measurable goals, approaches, timelines, and _____.
    A. Medications
    B. Assignments
    C. Expectations
    D. References

11. Employees in which department typically have the most interaction with residents without having an assignment to perform direct care services?
    A. Housekeeping
    B. Medical records
    C. Business office
    D. Maintenance

12. The consumer-oriented philosophy of senior care that emphasizes the importance of building services around consumer needs, expectations, and autonomy is broadly known as _____.
    A. Person-centered care
    B. Quality assurance and performance improvement
    C. The Green House Project
    D. The Eden Alternative

13. Person-directed care builds on the concept of person-centered care by adding emphasis on the importance of soliciting, respecting, and honoring the perspectives of _____.
    A. Residents and their families
    B. Care recipients and regulators
    C. Older adults and those who serve them most directly
    D. Clients

14. The first "culture change step" in moving a senior living organization away from an institutional model is to adopt a _____ model of service.
    A. Pod house
    B. Transformational
    C. Sunbeam
    D. Pioneer

15. Consistently applying _____ in ways that nimbly and effectively strengthen customer satisfaction is a hallmark of a skilled health services executive.
    A. Judgment
    B. Regulations
    C. Feedback
    D. Decisions

16. When physical or mental chronic conditions advance to a point that limits or significantly reduces a person's ability to routinely perform their own activities of daily living, then the focus turns to acquiring appropriate supports and services that enhance safety, security, and _____.
    A. Affordability
    B. Access
    C. Satisfaction
    D. Comfort

17. Customer service metrics in senior living tend to focus on a person's senses of _____, dignity, life satisfaction, value, and self-worth.
    A. Comfort
    B. Humor
    C. Awareness
    D. Spirituality

18. The emergence of _____ is a prime example of the continuing shift in senior living toward a hospitality model construct.
    A. Adult day centers
    C. Money follows the person
    B. The Program of All-Inclusive Care for the Aging
    D. Person-centered care

19. Dining services are most likely to be evaluated by consumers based on taste, temperature, texture, portion, nutrition, and _____.
    A. Presentation
    B. Saltiness
    C. Sweetness
    D. Calorie content

20. Which of the following is *not* a critical design dimension of a meaningful consumer satisfaction survey?
    A. Redundancy
    B. Anonymity
    C. Frequency
    D. Length

21. Sharing information from a completed customer satisfaction survey with participants, staff, and other appropriate stakeholders should include reporting on the results, responsive action steps, and _____.
    A. Rate of participation
    B. The cost of improvements
    C. Progress toward completing the action steps
    D. Announcing the next survey

22. Annual employee turnover in America's assisted living communities has been estimated as _____.
    A. Under 50%
    B. Between 35% and 55%
    C. Over 100%
    D. Over 70%

23. In order to most effectively schedule the optimal level of caregiving staff needed to meet the needs of the people they are serving, an assisted living community should know _____.
    A. Its current case mix
    B. The number of new hires in orientation
    C. Its overtime pay risk
    D. The average age of available staff

24. The employee acknowledgment included in a job description should establish that they understand its content as well as agree to perform the duties described and to _____.
    A. Accept the consequences of noncompliance
    B. Abide by all applicable policies, procedures, laws, and regulations
    C. Report any observed instances of noncompliance by others
    D. Participate in the performance evaluation process

25. If Olive Hill Assisted Living Community had an annualized employee turnover rate in the past year of 42%, then what was the retention rate for the same period?
    A. 58%
    B. 42%
    C. 142%
    D. 84%

26. The National Association of Long Term Care Administrator Boards has developed standards for minimum knowledge and skills to enter the profession, as well as for approving _____, accrediting academic programs in long-term care administration, and other regulatory guidelines to enhance its members' ability to meet their public protection charge.
    A. Licensure renewal
    B. Complaint investigations
    C. Continuing education
    D. Background checks

27. The two states that first licensed administrators leading assisted living communities are _____.
    A. Idaho and Washington
    B. Virginia and Ohio
    C. Idaho and Iowa
    D. Idaho and Virginia

28. The two primary sources of capital for a proprietary assisted living provider organization are debt financing and _____ financing.
    A. Equity
    B. Bank
    C. Bond
    D. Insurance

29. A popular way for assisted living community employees to have an ownership interest in their organization is called _____.
    A. A blind pool investment fund
    B. A risk-share entity (RSE)
    C. An investment opportunity employer (IOE)
    D. An employee stock ownership plan

30. The majority of contributions to a not-for-profit assisted living provider come from _____.
    A. Corporations
    B. Foundations
    C. Individuals
    D. Government grants

31. The dominant payer source for most assisted living communities is _____.
    A. Medicare Part A
    B. Privately paying consumers
    C. Medicaid
    D. Commercial long-term care insurance

32. The functions of a strong risk management program in the assisted living community setting include identification of methods to mitigate risk exposure, recognition of environmental and occupational risk exposures, application of risk control techniques to reduce errors and increase resident safety, and _____.
    A. Negotiation of favorable coverage terms with an insurance carrier
    B. Utilization of quality improvement techniques and tools
    C. Effective reservation of funds needed to cover anticipated liability losses
    D. Periodic quantification of the value of corporate assets

33. The most relevant key performance indicators to include in a senior living organization's dashboard are typically occupancy/census, revenues and expenses, staffing, client satisfaction and employee engagement, sales and marketing activity, and _____.
    A. Regulatory compliance and legislative initiatives
    B. Competitive forces and reimbursement changes
    C. Community image and employee retention
    D. Regulatory compliance and competitive forces

34. The _____ includes standards that set the foundation for electrical safety in residential, commercial, and industrial occupancies, including requirements for electrical wiring, overcurrent protection, grounding, and installation of equipment.
    A. National Electric Code
    B. North American Electrical Standards
    C. Life Safety Code (National Fire Protection Association-101 [NFPA-101])
    D. National Electrical Installation Standards

35. _____ is a planned activity designed to improve the performance and life of building systems or equipment, as well as to avoid mishaps requiring corrective interventions.
    A. Risk management
    B. Preventive maintenance
    C. Physical plant optimization
    D. Property stewardship

36. The National Fire Protection Association's (NFPA's) Life Safety Code illustrates the importance of proactively ensuring a _____ setting for people to live, work, and visit.
    A. Safe
    B. Secure
    C. Protected
    D. Contemporary

37. Regularly accounting for the arrival, storage, internal distribution, and reordering of supplies to ensure that there is enough of every product on hand when needed, and that any items with published expiration dates or shelf life are used within the prescribed time, is known as _____.
    A. Stock rotation
    B. Goods management
    C. Chain of custody
    D. Inventory control

38. Information that should be prominently and legibly displayed on a container that has been opened and stored, as well as food that has been prepared and saved for future serving, includes date, time, contents, and _____.
    A. When to use by or dispose
    B. Reheating temperature
    C. The name of the person completing the label
    D. Replacement order date

39. A "proprietary" senior living provider organization strives to generate an operational profit that benefits the ownership—typically _____.
    A. An individual
    B. A partnership
    C. An individual, partnership, or corporation
    D. A corporation

40. If a contracted therapy company's employee makes a harmful mistake, it is viewed as _____.
    A. A shared responsibility
    B. An extension of the provider organization
    C. The contractor's responsibility
    D. A breach of contract

41. The U.S. Department of Housing and Urban Development program that provides the very-low-income older adult population with options that allow them to live independently but with available supportive services—the Supportive Housing for the Elderly Program—is authorized in section _____ of the Housing and Urban Development Act.
    A. 202
    B. 1199
    C. A
    D. 501(c)(3)

42. The Malcolm Baldrige National Quality Award's criteria center on five key areas of outcome: product, process, or service; customer; leadership and governance; financial and market; and _____.
    A. Compliance
    B. Social impact
    C. Innovation
    D. Workforce

43. For a resident agreement to be legally enforceable, it typically must include provisions for mutual assent, consideration or exchange, absence of any element that violates the law, and _____.
    A. The capacity or competence of the parties making the agreement
    B. Disclosure of each party's full legal name
    C. Notary public's signature attestation
    D. The original agreement printed as a hard copy

44. In addition to learning about work design, conflict resolution, performance evaluation, communication styles, problem-solving methodologies, and coaching, a health services executive's preparation should include how to use tools for generating innovative ideas, building group consensus, fostering quality assurance and performance improvement, and _____.
    A. Managing inventory control
    B. Conducting effective meetings
    C. Coordinating staff scheduling
    D. Designing career ladder programs

45. Rather than identifying right answers or wrong answers, innovative leadership's primary goal is to _____.
    A. Refine and apply the success of others
    B. Reduce costs, increase revenues, or both
    C. Explore multiple possibilities and find a better solution
    D. Avoid recreating the wheel

46. What is the name of the national association that represents assisting living providers and has developed a specific sales counselor certificate program?
    A. LeadingAge
    B. American Health Care Association
    C. National Association of Long Term Care Administrator Boards
    D. Argentum

47. What part of senior living typically has the longest sales cycle?
    A. Senior housing community
    B. Skilled nursing facility
    C. Home care services
    D. Assisted living community

48. Which of the following is an example of a lead measure of organizational performance in an assisted living community?
    A. Annual employee turnover
    B. Call light response time
    C. Net operating margin
    D. Days cash on hand

49. _____ became one of the first states to license assisted living administrators in 2008, and its initial requirements have served as a model template for other licensing boards pursuing a similar path.
    A. Colorado
    B. Florida
    C. Virginia
    D. Oregon

50. The leading professional association representing the interests of providing training for senior housing managers is the _____.
    A. Department for Housing and Urban Development
    B. American College of Multi-Family Housing Directors
    C. National Center for Housing Management
    D. National Housing Investment Corporation

CHAPTER 10

Home- and Community-Based Services Practice Exam

1. The Centers for Medicare & Medicaid Services developed as the centerpiece of its Home Health Quality Reporting Program a patient assessment tool for evaluating people receiving skilled nursing care at home, which is the _____.
   A. Minimum Data Set
   B. Outcome and Assessment Information Set
   C. Prospective payment series
   D. Diagnostic-related grouping

2. The importance of spiritual wellness tends to _____ with advancing age.
   A. Increase
   B. Decline
   C. Remain constant
   D. Broaden

3. _____ of the states participate in the Nurse Licensure Compact, enabling nurses to practice in multiple states without having to obtain additional licenses.
   A. Fewer than one half
   B. Over two thirds
   C. Between one half and two thirds
   D. Between one third and one half

4. The standard credential awarded to someone who has met all the requirements to become an occupational therapist for a home health agency or hospice is _____.
   A. Licensed occupational therapist
   B. Registered occupational therapist
   C. Occupational therapist—registered and licensed
   D. Occupational therapist—qualified and registered

5. The health professional relied on to assess, diagnose, and treat communica-
   tion and swallowing disorders in a home- and community-based services
   setting is licensed by each state as a/an _____.
   A. Audiologist
   B. Speech and hearing technologist
   C. Otolaryngology therapist
   D. Speech language pathologist

6. A top barrier to providing most older adults living at home with routine den-
   tal treatment is _____.
   A. Poor oral hygiene habits
   B. Proximity to a dental office
   C. Low Medicaid reimbursement
   D. Access to transportation

7. The interdisciplinary team has as its core purpose developing a compre-
   hensive plan of care with clearly stated and _____ goals, approaches,
   timelines, and assignments.
   A. Measurable
   B. Succinct
   C. Evidence-based
   D. Adjustable

8. The consumer-oriented philosophy of senior care that emphasizes the im-
   portance of building services around consumer needs, expectations, and
   _____ is broadly known as person-centered care.
   A. Autonomy
   B. Safety
   C. Compliance
   D. Satisfaction

9. Person-_____ care builds on the concept of person-centered care by
   adding emphasis on the importance of soliciting, respecting, and honoring
   the perspectives of older adults and those who serve them most directly.
   A. Requested
   B. Sensitive
   C. Directed
   D. To-person

10. The _____ assessment form is completed for each home care recipient
    upon admission and periodically thereafter.
    A. Individual Service Plan
    B. Outcome and Assessment Information Set
    C. Minimum Data Set
    D. Patient Assessment Instrument

11. A Medicare-certified home health agency uses a client assessment tool referred to as the _____.
    A. Outcome and Assessment Information Set
    B. Patient Assessment Instrument
    C. Minimum Data Set
    D. Individual Service Plan

12. The central goal of the Improving Medicare Post-Acute Care Transformation Act was to achieve better health outcomes for Medicare beneficiaries through shared decision-making, enhanced discharge planning, and _____.
    A. Seamless transitions across the care continuum
    B. Reducing preventable rehospitalizations
    C. Eliminating surprise billing
    D. Effective care coordination

13. The Centers for Medicare & Medicaid Services' Five-Star Quality Rating System posted on its Home Health Compare website includes three major components: process metric, outcome metrics, and _____.
    A. Staffing
    B. Patient survey
    C. Compliance record
    D. Quality measures

14. Consistently applying feedback in ways that nimbly and effectively strengthen _____ is a hallmark of a skilled health services executive.
    A. Customer satisfaction
    B. Organizational depth
    C. Confidence
    D. Image

15. When physical or mental _____ conditions advance to a point that limits or significantly reduces a person's ability to routinely perform their own activities of daily living, then the focus turns to acquiring appropriate supports and services that enhance safety, security, and comfort.
    A. Stress
    B. Family
    C. Chronic
    D. Acute

16. Someone who receives care from a home health agency is most commonly called a _____.
    A. Participant
    B. Customer
    C. Patient
    D. Resident

17. A person served by an adult day center's programs is referred to as a
_____.

    A. Patient
    B. Participant
    C. Patron
    D. Resident

18. The overriding emphasis of _____ is postacute care, in contrast with the
acute care health system's primary objective of _____ a disease or repairing an injury.

    A. Aging services, preventing
    B. Human services, treating
    C. Transitional care, eliminating
    D. Senior living, curing

19. Hospice care strives to nurture a person's emotional, mental, and spiritual
needs on terms they express as important, not necessarily as dictated by the
_____.

    A. Regulations
    B. Cultural norms
    C. Provider
    D. Family

20. A critical design dimension of a meaningful consumer satisfaction survey is
_____.

    A. Ambiguity
    B. Anonymity
    C. Frequency
    D. Length

21. Sharing information from a completed customer satisfaction survey with participants, staff, and other appropriate stakeholders should include reporting
on the results, _____, and progress toward completing the action steps.

    A. Responsive action steps
    B. The cost of improvements
    C. Rate of participation
    D. Announcing the next survey

22. Annual employee turnover among home health agencies in America is estimated to be _____.

    A. Under 50%
    B. Over 70%
    C. Over 60%
    D. Between 35% and 55%

23. The collective scope and intensity of a home- and community-based senior living organization's customers is referred to as its _____.
    A. Recipient profile
    B. Cross-section score
    C. Care demand index
    D. Case mix

24. The employee acknowledgment included in a job description should establish that they _____, agree to perform the duties described, and accept the consequences of non-compliance.
    A. Understand its content
    B. Will report any observed instances of non-compliance by others
    C. Promise to participate in the performance evaluation process
    D. Pledge to abide by all applicable policies, procedures, laws, and regulations

25. It is important to clearly define in the employee handbook how expenses qualify for reimbursement, the process to follow for approval, and _____.
    A. The tax implications of receiving reimbursement
    B. Whether sales tax is recognized
    C. How to submit a request for reimbursement
    D. When the period for submitting expires

26. The Centers for Medicare & Medicaid Services requires Medicare- and Medicaid-certified long-term care providers to electronically submit _____ care staffing information called a Payroll-Based Journal.
    A. Comprehensive
    B. Direct
    C. Indirect
    D. Professional

27. In most states, the administrator of an organization that primarily provides home- and community-based services is required to have which credential from the following list?
    A. Nursing home administrator license
    B. Bachelor's degree in a health profession or business
    C. Health services executive qualification
    D. None of the above

28. Only one senior living service line has at least one half of its providers owned or sponsored by a not-for-profit organization: _____.
    A. Adult day centers
    B. Skilled nursing facilities
    C. Hospices
    D. Home health agencies

29. The evaluation and quality reporting system for home care that measures a person's condition and needs, which drives Medicare reimbursement, is known as the _____.
   A. Minimum Data Set
   B. Report on Optimal Assessment Data Statistics
   C. Outcome and Assessment Information Set
   D. Home Health Evaluation Tool

30. The Medicare-A home health Prospective Payment System includes payment for a 60-day episode, which can be renewed based on the person's _____.
   A. Maximum lifetime allowance
   B. Status regarding the Medicare "doughnut hole"
   C. Age
   D. Condition

31. The Medicare-A home health Prospective Payment System includes adjustments for _____ using the Outcome and Assessment Information Set categories.
   A. Staff travel time
   B. Case mix
   C. Primary diagnosis
   D. Care venue

32. Medicare consolidated billing for home health care requires a provider to bundle the costs for all services in a comprehensive rate, with the exception of _____.
   A. Durable medical equipment
   B. Transportation
   C. Disposable medical supplies
   D. Over-the-counter medications

33. Medicare's Patient-Driven Grouping Model for home healthcare relies on clinical characteristics and other patient information to define periods of care, and it eliminates the previous use of _____.
   A. A case mix index
   B. Actuarial tables
   C. Therapy service thresholds
   D. Resource utilization groups

34. Vehicle fleet management is a key risk avoidance and safety responsibility that should be considered _____.
   A. An indispensable expense
   B. A luxury
   C. A hidden cost
   D. An investment rather than a cost

35. Insurance carriers typically adjust premiums for covering company-owned or-leased vehicles based primarily on the _____.
    A. Driving record of those authorized to drive them
    B. Make and model of each vehicle
    C. Ages and health profiles of the passengers
    D. Grade of fuel each vehicle requires

36. The primary goal of an effective security program is to _____.
    A. Balance safety concerns with personal rights
    B. Minimize the risk of harm by outside forces
    C. Protect capital assets from avoidable damage
    D. Deter prospective intruders

37. When a care recipient who is incapable of adequately protecting themselves departs the premises unsupervised and undetected, it is known as _____.
    A. An escape
    B. A reportable event
    C. An elopement
    D. A Silver Alert

38. A not-for-profit or nonprofit senior living entity, formed to serve a community or members of a religious group or fraternal order, is often recognized by the U.S. Department of the Treasury's Internal Revenue Service as a _____ organization.
    A. Donor-supported
    B. Tax-free
    C. Community service
    D. Tax-exempt

39. An example of a public health service provider is _____.
    A. A home- and community-based service agency with a Medicaid waiver
    B. A Housing and Urban Development (HUD) Section 202 congregate housing complex
    C. A Medicare-certified home health agency
    D. The Department of Veterans Affairs

40. The federal agency that was originally created by the Older Americans Act and oversees a wide array of home- and community-based service programs through a national network of state Area Agencies on Aging and tribal organizations is currently known as the _____.
    A. National Council on Aging
    B. Administration on Community Living
    C. Administration on Aging
    D. Older Americans Agency

41. The agency within the U.S. Department of Health and Human Services that has overall responsibility for regulating postacute care providers that accept federal payments under either Title 18 or 19 of the Social Security Act is known as the _____.
    A. Social Security Administration
    B. Centers for Medicare & Medicaid Services
    C. Supplemental Security Income Agency
    D. Department of Housing and Urban Development

42. If a state wishes to offer health services that go beyond the minimum required by Medicaid, it may request special permission, called a _____, from the Centers for Medicare & Medicaid Services (CMS) to do so under section _____ of the Social Security Act's Title 19.
    A. Waiver, 1115
    B. Disclaimer, 1115
    C. Waiver, 1915
    D. Bond, 1215

43. In a civil lawsuit successfully brought against a home health agency, the three major categories of legal damages that can be awarded to the plaintiff are called nominal, compensatory, and _____ damages.
    A. Court cost
    B. Civil liability
    C. Punitive
    D. Statutory

44. It is imperative for a health services executive to develop and foster an organizational culture that portrays a core _____.
    A. Expectation of compliance
    B. Sense of caring
    C. Attention to detail
    D. Reliance on interdisciplinary teams

45. Identifying potential relationships that can strategically help fulfill a home healthcare provider's mission may include exploring new delivery systems, programs and services, or _____.
    A. Employees
    B. Vendors
    C. Stakeholders
    D. Markets

46. Which senior living service line generally has the shortest sales cycle?
    A. Adult day center
    B. Assisted living community
    C. Skilled nursing facility
    D. Senior housing community

47. A home- and community-based services organization's comprehensive approach aimed at influencing consumers' purchasing decisions is known as _____.
    A. Promotion
    B. Marketing
    C. Public relations
    D. Closing techniques

48. When public funds are accessed by provider organizations, there is a direct correlation with an expectation of quality oversight and a push toward greater transparency, such as the _____ program.
    A. Centers for Medicare & Medicaid Services' Five-Star Quality Rating System
    B. Joint Commission Accreditation
    C. U.S. News & World Report's Ratings
    D. American Health Care Association/National Center for Assisted Living's Quality Award

49. The core senior living leadership competencies are organized by the National Association of Long Term Care Administrator Boards into five categories, called domains of practice, and most of the academic preparation, _____, and continuing education programming in the field utilize this classification system.
    A. Experience
    B. Examinations
    C. Requirements
    D. Qualifications

50. Although licensure is required uniformly across all states and jurisdictions only for nursing home administrators, a voluntary, three-level, proficiency-based credential for a hospice organization's executive leader is available through the National Hospice and Palliative Care Organization's _____ program.
    A. Professional Certification
    B. Advanced Professional Management
    C. Palliative Care Management Competencies
    D. Hospice Management Development

PART III

Practice Exam Answers and Brief Rationales

CHAPTER 11

Answers + Brief Rationales for Core of Knowledge

1. Answer: **A.** Gerontology is the study of human aging, the most relevant and applicable discipline listed for a career in leading an organization serving predominantly older adults.

2. Answer: **D.** Interoperability means the ability of health information systems to work together within and across organizational boundaries in order to advance the effective delivery of healthcare for individuals and communities.

3. Answer: **B.** A clinical interdisciplinary team is typically led by a physician and concentrates on assessing the health needs of care recipients and developing and delivering a plan of care; a support services interdisciplinary team is comprised of staff members from nonclinical disciplines whose efforts complement the clinical team.

4. Answer: **B.** According to the National Institutes of Health, diseases of the cardiovascular system—heart failure, coronary artery disease, and atrial fibrillation—are the most common reasons for health visits and hospital stays experienced by older adults.

5. Answer: **A.** Crystalized intelligence refers to knowledge gained through education and experience; acquired intelligence is a synonym for crystalized intelligence; calculating refers to manipulation and interpretation of data.

6. Answer: **D.** Crystalized intelligence refers to knowledge gained through education and experience.

7. Answer: **C.** According to the Centers for Disease Control and Prevention, depression is associated with distress and suffering, and it also can lead to impairments in physical, mental, and social functioning, often complicating the treatment of other chronic diseases.

8. Answer: **A.** Each of the other response options relates to technology, but health information technology is the only option that encompasses all of the elements of this definition.

9. Answer: **A.** None of the alternate response options is the name of an actual congressional act.

10. Answer: **D.** Health Level Seven International has over 1,600 members from over 50 countries representing healthcare providers, government agencies, vendors, payers, vendors, and suppliers.

11. Answer: **C.** While each of the alternate response options is a possible outcome of the Health Information Technology for Economic and Clinical Health Act's implementation, none of them were core goals of the legislation.

12. Answer: **A.** A physical therapist now requires a doctoral degree, the doctorate of physical therapy. The DPT is a clinical degree, also referred to as a professional degree, whereas other doctoral degrees (PhD, EdD, etc.) are academic degrees not limited to any one discipline or profession.

13. Answer: **D.** The American Podiatric Medical Association reports that older patients most commonly complain to its members about toe deformities, nail conditions, calluses, and corns.

14. Answer: **A.** The Centers for Disease Control and Prevention's list of the most frequently diagnosed and treated vision conditions among older Americans begins with cataracts.

15. Answer: **B.** The alternate response options could each be contributory to the field of health informatics.

16. Answer: **C.** Universal and body substance isolation procedures are precursors to standard precautions; contact precaution procedures are typically applied in addition to standard precautions.

17. Answer: **D.** Over 80% of nursing home residents need help with three or more activities of daily living; about 90% of residents who are able to walk need assistance or supervision.

18. Answer: **B.** The World Health Organization defines "acute care" as the treatment of sudden, often unexpected, urgent, or emergent episodes of injury and illness that can lead to death or disability without rapid intervention. Senior living lines of service sometimes overlap with or complement this realm but place greater emphasis on enhancing quality of life and contentment.

19. Answer: **A.** A power differential is the inherently greater power and influence that helping professionals have as compared with the people they help. Understanding both the value and the many impacts of the power differential is the core of ethical awareness.

20. Answer: **D.** Supported by Doty, M. M., Koren, M. J., & Sturla, E. L. (2008, May). *Culture change in nursing homes: How far have we come? Findings from the Commonwealth Fund National Survey of Nursing Homes. The Commonwealth Fund.* www.commonwealthfund.org/publications/fund-reports/2008/may/culture -change-nursing-homes-how-far-have-we-come-findings

21. Answer: **C.** Former TV news anchor Tom Brokaw coined the terms in his best-selling book *The Greatest Generation.*

22. Answer: **B.** The discussion relevant to the answer can be explained in the following references: Brokaw, T. (1998). *The greatest generation.* Random House. Dychtwald, K., & Croker, R. (2009). *Boomer Century: 1946 -2046: How America's most influential generation changed everything.* Grand Central Publishing.

23. Answer: **B.** The alternate response choices duplicate one of the elements in the question's stem.

24. Answer: **D.** The elements included in the question's stem really do not matter much to the consumer if the person providing services is not readily and consistently available.

25. Answer: **C.** It is paramount that a provider communicates with consumers and their representatives in ways that they understand.

26. Answer: **A.** Protecting one's privacy includes keeping information about them confidential.

27. Answer: **C.** This is a fundamental premise of the Health Insurance Portability and Accountability Act.

28. Answer: **D.** This is the most comprehensive response option.

29. Answer: **C.** This ultimate question has shown to be an effective measure of overall satisfaction.

30. Answer: **B.** It is essential to go beyond "talking the talk" of innovation and weave creativity into the organization's culture, leading by example and "walking the walk."

31. Answer: **A.** Occupations involving the personal care of people and having access to sensitive personal information may leave felons out due to their criminal record; working in the senior living field requires honesty and ethical behavior.

32. Answer: **A.** An agreement takes an offer and an acceptance.

33. Answer: **D.** The Internal Revenue Service requires every employer that pays remuneration for services performed by an employee to have each employee complete Form W-4 so that the employer can withhold the correct federal income tax from the employee's pay.

34. Answer: **C.** The Internal Revenue Service requires every employer to have each employee complete Form I-9 to verify the identity and employment authorization of individuals hired for employment in the United States; the employee must also present their employer with acceptable documents evidencing identity and employment authorization.

35. Answer: **C.** Self-directed work teams, which originally surfaced in manufacturing, have been successfully introduced in service industries such as senior living.

36. Answer: **B.** The alternate response options address policies or procedures of the organization; this response is part of the job requirements.

37. Answer: **D.** The U.S. Department of Labor's Wage and Hour Division describes the regulations promulgated following the enactment of the Family Medical Leave Act, available at www.dol.gov/agencies/whd/fmla.

38. Answer: **A.** The Internal Revenue Service holds that an essential element of a de minimis benefit is that it is occasional or unusual in frequency.

39. Answer: **A.** The Fair Labor Standards Act's (FLSA) exempt status refers to the state of being exempt from the protection provided by the FLSA concerning overtime eligibility requirements; employers are typically not required to pay overtime to employees with the listed responsibilities.

40. Answer: **B.** Retention of employees is generally a systemic effort supported by human resources; the alternate response choices are tied more closely to either departmental supervisors (scheduling and evaluating performance) or financial management (paying).

41. Answer: **C.** These are necessary to perform the services expected from the practitioner; the alternate response options can certainly prove beneficial but are not as essential as knowledge and skills of the discipline.

42. Answer: **D.** According to The Federation of Associations of Regulatory Boards, expecting licensed professionals to engage in some form of structured lifelong learning about their discipline's best practices and current evidence-based standards of care is the norm across the spectrum of health professions.

43. Answer: **A.** In addition to showing up for work, it is important for a staff member to actively engage in the delivery of care and services in order to fulfill the organization's mission.

44. Answer: **B.** According to the U.S. Bureau of Labor Statistics, the absence rate among staff members of senior living organizations is estimated to be 10%.

45. Answer: **A.** While human resources may play an advisory role in each of the alternate response options, it is most likely to be engaged in the hiring process.

46. Answer: **D.** This is a description of an income statement according to generally accepted accounting principles, which are set forth by the Financial Accounting Standards Board.

47. Answer: **C.** This is a description of a balance sheet according to generally accepted accounting principles, which are set forth by the Financial Accounting Standards Board.

48. Answer: **D.** This is a description of a cash flow statement according to generally accepted accounting principles, which are set forth by the Financial Accounting Standards Board.

49. Answer: **A.** The alternate response options do not reflect an organization's profitability.

50. Answer: **C.** Debt service coverage =

    (Annual income available for debt payments)

    (Annual principal + Interest payments)

51. Answer: **C.** Variable expenses are tied to fluctuations in census, revenues, or expenses (such as staffing or supplies), and fixed expenses typically remain constant (such as a mortgage).

52. Answer: **A.** A capital purchase is a large amount (an organization determines the threshold, typically $1,000–5,000), and it acquires an asset with a useful life of more than 1 year.

53. Answer: **D.** Each of the alternate response options duplicates one of the capital financing options included in the question.

54. Answer: **B.** A Medicare Advantage Plan operates similarly to a health maintenance organization and is offered by private insurance companies approved by Medicare in lieu of Medicare A and B.

55. Answer: **A.** Medicare Part A covers the services listed in the question and is typically provided at no additional cost for eligible enrollees.

56. Answer: **A.** Medicare Part B is medical insurance that covers a wide range of services, supplies, and equipment separate from hospital care.

57. Answer: **A.** The easiest way to remember which kind of benefits are covered by Medicare Part D is that "D" is the first letter of the word "Drugs."

58. Answer: **C.** Answer supported by a study by Stevenson, Cohen, Tell, and Burwell. Stevenson, D. G., Cohen, M. A., Tell, E. J., & Burwell, B. (2010). The complementarity of public and private long-term care coverage. *Health Affairs, 29*(1), 96–101.

59. Answer: **A.** Cybersecurity is the protection of internet-based systems, including hardware, software, and data, from cyberattacks. In a computing context, security comprises cybersecurity and physical security—both are used by enterprises to protect against unauthorized access to data centers and other computerized systems.

60. Answer: **A.** An annual report typically includes an independent auditor's report; a social impact statement goes beyond an organization's financial performance and reports on how its operation has benefited the community it serves; financial performance verification is a fictional term.

61. Answer: **D.** The first response is a fictitious substitute for the Federal Emergency Management Agency. The National Council on Building Codes and Standards (NCBCS) is a unit of the National Institute of Building Sciences, the federal agency that serves as the authoritative voice supporting advances in building science and technology to improve the built environment. Architects must follow the safety guidelines set forth by the National Fire Protection Association (NFPA) in designing new buildings or modifying existing structures, with unique provisions for residential occupancy and the provision of healthcare services.

62. Answer: **A.** The NFPA-101 standard addresses construction, protection, and occupancy features necessary to minimize danger to life from the effects of fire, including smoke, heat, and toxic gases created during a fire.

63. Answer: **B.** Each of the alternate response options could occur but only in the event that the correct response precedes it.

64. Answer: **A.** The goal of computer redundancy is to prevent—or recover from—the failure of a specific component of the system; the most common form of computer redundancy is a backup storage device.

65. Answer: **C.** Understanding the organization's prospects for responding effectively is the most critical element listed among the response options.

66. Answer: **C.** An active aggressor can appear in any location.

67. Answer: **D.** Size is the only response option that is a product specification.

68. Answer: **C.** Each of the alternate response options either cites an irrelevant part of the IRS code or follows an improper rubric.

69. Answer: **B.** Only a governmental agency has the authority to issue a license to practice a health profession; certification of advanced proficiency in a discipline or procedure may be awarded by private organizations.

70. Answer: **A.** A suit in response to an event that results in personal injury and a landlord–tenant dispute are examples of a civil action.

71. Answer: **C.** In order to compete successfully, going beyond the minimum requirements is a well-established strategy for prevailing in the marketplace.

72. Answer: **A.** One manages systems and things but leads people.

73. Answer: **C.** Managers keep the organization's motor running, and leaders plot the course for where to travel.

74. Answer: **A.** Answer is supported by the following: Jago, A. G. (1982). Leadership: Perspectives in theory and research. *Management Science, 28*(3), 315–337.

75. Answer: **D.** Answer is supported by the following: Bass, B. A. (1996). *A new paradigm of leadership: An inquiry into transformational leadership.* U.S. Army Research Institute for the Behavioral and Social Sciences.

76. Answer: **D.** A person's emotional intelligence quotient is a measure of their depth, breadth, and balance across the four quadrants, including how effectively one manages relationships.

77. Answer: **B.** In order to fully apply the other characteristics listed in the question's stem, it is essential for a servant leader to be seen regularly and perceived as engaged and approachable.

78. Answer: **C.** The Multifactor Leadership Questionnaire was developed by Bass and Avoliio over 20 years ago; numerous studies have validated its use as a tool for measuring the personal influence of leaders.

79. Answer: **A.** At the center of the Leadership Practices Inventory is the weight placed on a leader's effectiveness in advocating for a vision of a better tomorrow.

80. Answer: **D.** It is not enough to be a proficient provider of needed services in today's senior living field; considering the needs of the different stakeholders and conveying a genuine concern for the well-being of others especially in senior care must be woven into the very fabric of the organization's culture. The organization's values should be in alignment with those of the people it serves.

81. Answer: **C.** Assessing an organization's strengths and weaknesses helps inform its view of both its opportunities and its threats.

82. Answer: **B.** The Plan–Do–Check–Act cycle was introduced first in a manufacturing context; it is sometimes also referred to as the Deming or Shewhart circle, cycle, or wheel after the engineers who proposed, applied, and refined the model.

83. Answer: **D.** "Begin with the end in mind" is one of Dr. Covey's 7 Habits of Highly Effective People. Covey, S. R. (1989). *The seven habits of highly effective people: Restoring the character ethic.* Simon and Schuster.

84. Answer: **A.** Answers the questions, "What? How? Who? Possible? and When?"

85. Answer: **C.** As operational variation decreases, so does uncertainty and rework.

86. Answer: **D.** People must have confidence in their leader's integrity and competence in order to enthusiastically follow them.

87. Answer: **D.** Lewin's three-step model of organizational change includes unfreezing, moving, and refreezing (stabilization).

88. Answer: **A.** Lippett's model of organizational change envisions the use of a change agent to help the organization navigate the process, as well as the cyclical nature of change.

89. Answer: **A.** Top-of-mind awareness refers to the status of a brand—service or product—as the first one a potential customer thinks about when asked to consider a particular industry.

90. Answer: **B.** The four Ps of marketing are product, price, promotion, and place.

91. Answer: **C.** Each of the alternate response options represents some form of service identification but not necessarily an external–internal comparison.

92. Answer: **B.** Critical thinking is the intellectually disciplined process of actively and skillfully conceptualizing, applying, analyzing, synthesizing, and/or evaluating information gathered from, or generated by, observation, experience, reflection, reasoning, or communication, as a guide to belief and action.

93. Answer: **A.** The DECIDE model, introduced by Guo (2008) for healthcare managers to apply in their decision-making, stands for the following: define the problem; establish the criteria; consider all alternatives; identify the best alternative; develop and implement an action plan; and evaluate and monitor the solution and feedback. Guo, K. L. (2008). DECIDE: A decision-making model for more effective decision making by health care managers. *Health Care Management, 27*(2), 118–127. doi.org/10.1097/01 .HCM.0000285046.27290.90

94. Answer: **A.** The fishbone diagram (aka the Ishikawa diagram) is a cause-and-effect diagram that helps managers identify the reasons for imperfections, variations, defects, or failures. The diagram looks just like a fish's skeleton, with the problem at its head and the causes for the problem feeding into the spine.

95. Answer: **D.** A leadership dashboard facilitates measuring, monitoring, and managing the key activities and processes needed to achieve strategic goals.

96. Answer: **B.** Goals, objectives, and tactics are each subsets or components of strategy.

97. Answer: **A.** Six Sigma is an operational improvement model.

98. Answer: **C.** Licensure by equivalency describes accepting a standard that meets or exceeds the state's licensure regulations concerning qualifications, knowledge, and skills.

99. Answer: **D.** Since 1962, the American College of Health Care Administrators has been a non-profit professional membership association dedicated to representing and serving individual professionals in long-term care administration and the postacute care arena.

100. Answer: **A.** A professional development plan requires an individual to reflect on their strength and growth areas and take ownership of their own development.

CHAPTER 12

Answers + Brief Rationales for Nursing Home Administration

1. Answer: **B.** None of the third-party programs listed require input from a dietary manager, head chef, or culinary expert.

2. Answer: **A.** The American Medical Directors Association officially changed its name in 2014 to The Society for Post-Acute and Long-Term Care Medicine.

3. Answer: **C.** The Centers for Medicare & Medicaid Services combines the terms "quality assurance" and "performance improvement" to describe taking a systematic, comprehensive, and data-driven approach to maintaining and improving safety and quality in nursing homes while involving residents, families, and all nursing home caregivers in practical and creative problem-solving.

4. Answer: **B.** The key word in the question's stem is "effective"; the alternate response options each describe a positive outcome—but not efficacy.

5. Answer: **B.** A clinical interdisciplinary team is typically led by a physician and concentrates on assessing the health needs of residents and developing and delivering a plan of care; a support services interdisciplinary team is comprised of staff members from nonclinical disciplines whose efforts complement those of the clinical team.

6. Answer: **D.** The Centers for Medicare & Medicaid Services (and most commercial payers) requires that a licensed medical doctor direct the overall care of a resident receiving services in a skilled nursing facility.

7. Answer: **D.** 42 CFR 483.70(h) requires that the medical director be a licensed physician.

8. Answer: **B.** 42 CFR 483.152(b) stipulates federally mandated course content for a training program to prepare someone to become a certified nurse aide.

9. Answer: **B.** The alternate response options are fictional credentials.

10. Answer: **D.** 42 CFR 483.15 requires a skilled nursing facility to provide "medically related social services to attain or maintain the highest practicable resident physical, mental and psychosocial well-being"; more than 120 beds require a full-time social worker with at least a bachelor's degree in the discipline.

11. Answer: **D.** The alternate response options are fictional organizations.

12. Answer: **B.** The Society for Post-Acute and Long-Term Care Medicine developed this credentialing program in collaboration with professional organizations representing the interests of physicians specializing in internal medicine, family practice, and geriatrics.

13. Answer: **C.** As part of the Affordable Care Act, the Centers for Medicare & Medicaid Services was directed to launch a focus on quality best practices that would support improvements in long term care. They combined the terms "quality assurance" and "performance improvement" to describe taking a systematic, comprehensive, and data-driven approach to maintaining and improving safety and quality in nursing homes.

14. Answer: **D.** Life satisfaction is the only response option that is not a subset of one of the three issues included in the question stem; regulatory compliance and infection control are closely related to either safety or quality, and disaster preparedness is related to safety.

15. Answer: **B.** The Minimum Data Set is required by the Centers for Medicare & Medicaid Services for the skilled nursing facility setting.

16. Answer: **A.** The Minimum Data Set has 21 sections; all three of the other response options are section titles.

17. Answer: **B.** The Centers for Medicare & Medicaid Services inpatient rehabilitation facility quality reporting program describes the Patient Assessment Instrument; it expects Medicare-certified providers to utilize the program.

18. Answer: **C.** The Centers for Medicare & Medicaid Services' Nursing Home Quality Initiative Program describes the Minimum Data Set; it expects Medicare- and Medicaid-certified providers to utilize the program.

19. Answer: **A.** Although all of the alternative response options are important operational considerations, the fifth element the CMS expects a provider's quality assurance and performance improvement program to include concerns feedback, data systems, and monitoring.

20. Answer: **B.** The CMS's "Five-Star Quality Rating System" for skilled nursing facilities is described at www.cms.gov/Medicare/Provider-Enrollment-and-Certification/CertificationandComplianc/FSQRS.

21. Answer: **C.** It is essential to gather candid critiques from customers about their care experiences to inform decisions about resource allocations that can enhance performance.

22. Answer: **D.** Multiple studies have shown that employee turnover in skilled nursing facilities has consistently been about 75% annually.

23. Answer: **B.** The Institute of Medicine's Committee on Nursing Home Regulation published its first findings in 1986 and has periodically updated its recommendations based on the most contemporary evidence.

24. Answer: **D.** The Institute of Medicine's Committee on Nursing Home Regulation published its first findings in 1986 and has periodically updated its recommendations based on the most contemporary evidence.

25. Answer: **B.** Centers for Medicare & Medicaid Services' State Operations Manual for Long-Term Care Facilities participating in Medicare or Medicaid, based on 42 CFR 483 to attain or maintain the highest practicable well-being level for residents.

26. Answer: **D.** Section 6106 of the Affordable Care Act requires electronic submission of direct care staffing information (including agency and contract staff) based on payroll.

27. Answer: **A.** 42 CFR 431.700–7.15 amended the Social Security Act to require each state to include in its State Health Plan a board of licensure for nursing home administrators.

28. Answer: **C.** Per Title XIX of the Social Security Act, Medicaid has both a means (income and assets) test and a medical need requirement.

29. Answer: **B.** Eligibility for both programs requires a combination of age or disability and low-enough financial resources.

30. Answer: **D.** Although the percentage can vary somewhat by state, Medicaid is the leading source of reimbursement for skilled nursing facilities.

31. Answer: **A.** Equalization laws are an effective policy approach to the elimination of cross-subsidization. However, if the Medicaid level of payment is inadequate, then the range and quality of services all nursing home residents receive, not just Medicaid patients, would likely decline in a state using this equalization approach.

32. Answer: **B.** The Patient-Driven Payment Model actually replaces resource utilization groups with a base rate and case mix index. Diagnosis-related groups apply to acute care settings, and the Minimum Data Set is a resident assessment tool used primarily for care planning and/or resource allocation.

33. Answer: **C.** The implementation of the Patient-Driven Payment Model illustrates the move by the Centers for Medicare & Medicaid Services away from recognizing costs based on services provided and toward payment for services responding to identified resident needs.

34. Answer: **D.** NFPA-101 is not a regulation promulgated by a government agency but a set of standards that many government agencies with responsibilities for public safety rely on, including the Centers for Medicare & Medicaid Services.

35. Answer: **B.** The Health Insurance Portability and Accountability Act (HIPAA) administrative simplification rules require retaining a medical record for 6 years from the date of its creation or the date when it last was in effect, whichever is later; HIPAA requirements preempt any state law that requires a shorter period (45 CFR 164.316(b)(2)).

36. Answer: **C.** In 2008, any skilled nursing facility without a compliant sprinkler system and at least two separate areas with special fire-resistant building materials and fire-rated doors that wanted to continue in the Medicare and Medicaid programs was given until 2013 to complete the work.

37. Answer: **A.** The second-most cited deficiency is consistently food safety, and one of the four most common contributors to those findings is leftover food without a discard date.

38. Answer: **B.** Each of the alternate response options is a report on an external phenomenon.

39. Answer: **D.** 42 CFR 483, "Requirements for States and Long Term Care Facilities," is complemented by detailed instructions about compliance with the regulations in the State Operations Manual.

40. Answer: **D.** There is a category with the title, Quality of Life, which has elements addressing residents' levels of life satisfaction.

41. Answer: **B.** None of the alternate response options necessarily prompt a CMS/state compliance survey.

42. Answer: **A.** The purpose for visiting to observe is decidedly different between confirming minimal compliance with regulatory standards and recognizing performance beyond those standards. Arriving unannounced for a compliance survey enables the team to observe normal operations on any given day.

43. Answer: **D.** There is abundant evidence from studies about quality assurance and performance improvement models that have been effective in other fields to challenge the efficacy of the current regulatory enforcement system for long-term care facilities.

44. Answer: **B.** 42 CFR 431.700–7.15 amended the Social Security Act to require each state to include in its State Health Plan a board of licensure for nursing home administrators.

45. Answer: **B.** 42 CFR 431.700–7.15 amended the Social Security Act to require each state to include in its board of licensure for nursing home administrators persons with certain qualifications.

46. Answer: **A.** States followed the federal mandate to form licensing boards, but there were no guidelines or templates to follow; sharing information about board composition, policies and procedures, qualifications, and other operational high-impact practices was swiftly recognized as needed and desired.

47. Answer: **B.** "Administrator-in-Training" is the term of art that is most widely used in senior living leadership.

48. Answer: **D.** State nursing home administrator licensing regulations typically refer to the administrative mentor and supervisor for someone completing an "Administrator-in-Training" assignment as their preceptor.

49. Answer: **C.** Reciprocal means bidirectional; "We'll recognize your state's license in exchange for your state recognizing ours."

50. Answer: **B.** Endorsement signifies support or approval of another board's decision to issue a professional license but not necessarily with any expectation of mutual exchange.

CHAPTER 13

Answers + Brief Rationales for Residential Care and Assisted Living

1. Answer: **B.** Applied technology enhances a person's wellness, comfort, or safety; health information technology helps manage data to support health services operations.

2. Answer: **C.** The only senior living–related organization listed is the Pioneer Network.

3. Answer: **A.** The household model follows institutional, transformational, and neighborhood models in the sequence of stages referred to as "culture change" in senior living settings.

4. Answer: **B.** According to the Centers for Disease Control and Prevention, the leading causes of death among Americans aged 65 and over are as follows (in descending order): heart disease, cancer, chronic obstructive pulmonary disease, stroke, Alzheimer's disease, diabetes, pneumonia and flu, and accidents.

5. Answer: **C.** Each of the response options is plausible; avoiding disability and disease has the most powerful impact.

6. Answer: **A.** Research shows that religion and spirituality are seen by older adults as positive forces that help them face life with more resilience and hope, improve social and familial relationships, and cope with life stresses such as financial or health concerns.

7. Answer: **C.** The National Association of Activities Professionals includes such titles in its continuing education offerings and training materials.

8. Answer: **A.** Modern dentistry is typically equipment intensive and relies on specialized instruments that require routine sterilization, light radiology capability, and hazardous medical waste disposal; hence, service delivery is often limited to a fixed space, and patients with limited transportation options encounter dental care barriers related to their ability to appear in person.

9. Answer: **D.** A beautician, cosmetologist, barber, or nail care specialist typically has more focused time to socially interact with a resident while providing services than most other service providers, enabling them to observe (and report) any significant or abrupt changes in a resident's affect or behavior.

10. Answer: **B.** It is important to know who is responsible for carrying out the various components of the care plan developed by the team.

11. Answer: **A.** While employees from none of the listed departments typically perform direct care services, members of the housekeeping staff generally encounter residents at least daily.

12. Answer: **A.** Both the Green House Project and the Eden Alternative are branded forms of person-centered care; quality assurance and performance improvement is a systems monitoring and improvement method.

13. Answer: **C.** This is the most complete response of the options offered—"those who serve them most directly" can include family, friends, volunteers, or staff.

14. Answer: **B.** The Commonwealth Fund supported a study to examine the key elements of culture change, which identified four stages of development—institutional, transformational, neighborhood, and household models.

15. Answer: **C.** Customer-centered decisions typically win loyalty and enhance an organization's competitive position.

16. Answer: **D.** Protection from harm and discomfort are the two most pressing needs people have when their autonomy declines due to either diminishing cognitive capability or diminishing physical capability.

17. Answer: **A.** Comfort is a more basic and cherished parameter than any of the alternate response options.

18. Answer: **D.** Building programs and services around customer needs and preferences is a hallmark of person-centered care.

19. Answer: **A.** Saltiness and sweetness are taste metrics; calories are related to portion and nutrition. Presentation addresses appeal and attraction for consumption.

20. Answer: **B.** Redundancy or validation can strengthen the power of a satisfaction survey's results, but it is not as essential as protecting participants' anonymity, how often it is performed, or how long it takes for someone to complete it.

21. Answer: **C.** People generally want to know whether their participation in a satisfaction survey will lead to improvements and whether their input mattered.

22. Answer: **D.** Surveys by Argentum and McKnight's Long-Term Care support this response. Argentum. (2018). *Senior living labor and workforce trends: 2018 Forecasts.* Author. erickson.umbc.edu/files/2018/02/Argentum -Senior-Living-Labor-Workforce-Trends-2018.pdf; McKnight's Staff. (2012, October 16). Survey assesses turnover and retention rates among assist-ed living workers. McKnight's Long-Term Care News. www.mcknights .com/news/survey-assesses-turnover-and-retention-rates-among-assisted -living-workers/

23. Answer: **A.** Knowing the collective demand for service intensity (acuity of need) and scope (how many people have each level of need) is essential to assign staff resources to appropriately meet those needs.

24. Answer: **B.** Each of the alternate response options is a subset of the correct answer.

25. Answer: **A.** (Retention rate) + (turnover rate) = 100%.

26. Answer: **C.** The National Association of Long Term Care Administrator Boards' National Continuing Education Review Service reviews and approves thousands of continuing education (CE) programs offered by hundreds of CE providers.

27. Answer: **D.** Idaho began licensing administrators of assisted living facilities in 1993; Virginia followed suit in 2008.

28. Answer: **A.** Although the mix can vary somewhat regionally, debt and equity capital financing are the two dominant sources accessed nationally by devel-opers of assisted living communities.

29. Answer: **D.** The alternate response options are less plausible; a blind pool in-vestment fund would not necessarily include employees of the organization, and both the RSE and IOE are fictional acronyms.

30. Answer: **C.** Individuals are responsible for the majority of charitable giving in America.

31. Answer: **B.** According to the National Care Planning Council, family out-of-pocket funds account for the vast majority of revenues for assisted living communities.

32. Answer: **B.** The alternate response options are not preventive measures aimed at mitigating risk.

33. Answer: **D.** Mission and vision for the organization generally drive key per-formance indicators but regulatory compliance and competitive forces are the two additions to the list that are likely to have the greatest impact on its success.

34. Answer: **A.** Also known as NFPA-70, the National Electric Code is a companion set of standards to the NFPA-101; the North American Electrical Standards combines standards from the United States and Canada; National Electrical Installation Standards is a fictional entity.

35. Answer: **B.** An ounce of prevention is worth a pound of repairs; proactively scheduling routine checks on buildings and equipment typically fosters early detection of potential challenges ranging from business interruption to safety concerns.

36. Answer: **A.** NFPA-101 establishes standards for the design of a safe environment.

37. Answer: **D.** This is the most plausible response; stock rotation is an activity sometimes applied in an inventory control process; chain of custody addresses who has had control of an item from the time it leaves the manufacturer until it is used; goods management is a fabricated term.

38. Answer: **C.** The most critical additional piece of information for addressing any uncertainty about the contents of the container is who opened, resealed, and stored it.

39. Answer: **C.** A proprietary sponsorship can take the form of any of the response options.

40. Answer: **B.** It is possible to delegate authority to another entity but not to assign (and waive) responsibility.

41. Answer: **A.** This is the only section applicable to the referenced Act.

42. Answer: **D.** The award recognizes U.S. organizations in the business, healthcare, education, and nonprofit sectors for performance excellence; it is managed by the National Institute of Standards and Technology, an agency of the U.S. Department of Commerce.

43. Answer: **A.** Each party to a contract must possess the ability to comprehend what the agreement is about and its legal standing to make an autonomous decision.

44. Answer: **B.** Of the possible responses, the health services executive is most likely to be directly engaged in conducting meetings.

45. Answer: **C.** Exploring multiple possibilities to find a solid solution invites stakeholder engagement, as well as the prospect of a wider variety of possibilities from which to choose.

46. Answer: **D.** Formerly known as the Assisted Living Federation of America, the association rebranded in 2015 as Argentum (derived from the Latin word for "silver," intending to convey strength and a sense of gravitas while giving a nod to the silver generation).

47. Answer: **A.** Choosing a senior housing community is a lifestyle decision; the alternate response options are each driven more by needs for supportive services, relatively.

48. Answer: **B.** Call light response time is more directly related to specific performance in responding to residents' needs than any of the alternate response options.

49. Answer: **C.** Idaho began licensing administrators of assisted living facilities in 1993; Virginia followed suit in 2008.

50. Answer: **C.** The National Center for Housing Management is the only response option offered that is a professional association and offers training for senior housing managers.

CHAPTER 14

Answers + Brief Rationales for Home- and Community-Based Services

1. Answer: **B.** None of the other potential responses relate to the home health setting.

2. Answer: **A.** Research shows that religion and spirituality are seen by older adults as positive forces that help them face life with more resilience and hope, improve social and familial relationships, and cope with life stresses such as financial or health concerns.

3. Answer: **B.** The National Council of State Boards of Nursing lists 34 states as participating in the Nurse Licensure Compact.

4. Answer: **C.** The alternate response options are fictional credentials.

5. Answer: **D.** This is the only licensed health professional role matching the scope of practice described.

6. Answer: **D.** Modern dentistry is typically equipment intensive and relies on specialized instruments that require routine sterilization, light radiology capability, and hazardous medical waste disposal; hence, service delivery is often limited to a fixed space, and patients with limited transportation options encounter dental care barriers related to their ability to appear in person.

7. Answer: **A.** It is important to understand what is expected, by whom, and when for carrying out the various components of the care plan developed by the team.

8. Answer: **A.** Protecting and preserving one's autonomy is the hallmark of person-centered care.

9. Answer: **C.** Person-*directed* care attempts to put the care recipient in charge at every opportunity.

10. Answer: **B.** The Centers for Medicare & Medicaid Services requires the Outcome and Assessment Information Set for persons receiving skilled nursing care at home.

11. Answer: **A.** The Centers for Medicare & Medicaid Services' (CMS's) Home Health Quality Reporting Program describes the Outcome and Assessment Information Set; the CMS expects Medicare-certified providers to utilize it.

12. Answer: **D.** In 2014, HR 4994 was passed by Congress as Public Law 113-185 and signed by President Obama. It was designed to create a standardized platform for assessing treatment methods, quality measures, and health outcomes achieved by postacute care providers.

13. Answer: **B.** Home Health Compare is available at www.cms.gov/ Medicare/Quality-Initiatives-Patient-Assessment-Instruments/ HomeHealthQualityInits/HHQIHomeHealthStarRatings.

14. Answer: **A.** Customer-centered decisions typically win loyalty and enhance an organization's competitive position.

15. Answer: **C.** Protection from harm and discomfort are the two most pressing needs people have when their autonomy declines due to either diminishing cognitive capability or diminishing physical capability.

16. Answer: **C.** Although some organizations may refer to a care recipient as a "customer" or "consumer" to emphasize the business relationship, "patient" is the more commonly applied title for people receiving healthcare services in their own homes.

17. Answer: **B.** Although some adult day centers may refer to a care recipient as a "patient" due to the healthcare focus of the services rendered, the preferred title for a person participating in programs offered in this setting is "participant," intended to depict their active engagement.

18. Answer: **D.** The World Health Organization defines "acute care" as the treatment of sudden, often unexpected, urgent or emergent episodes of injury and illness that can lead to death or disability without rapid intervention. Senior living lines of service sometimes overlap with or complement this realm but place greater emphasis on enhancing quality of life and contentment.

19. Answer: **C.** The hospice movement inspired other segments of senior living and healthcare to replace provider-centered care (built for efficiency) with person-centered care (designed for consumer satisfaction).

20. Answer: **B.** Participation must be free of any fear of reprisal.

21. Answer: **A.** People generally want to know whether their participation in a satisfaction survey will lead to improvements and whether their input mattered.

22. Answer: **C.** A 2015 study published by PHI National's Direct Care Workforce Center found that home care worker turnover tops 60% annually. Scales, K. (2018). *Growing a strong direct care workforce: A recruitment and retention guide for employers*. PHI Direct Care Workforce Resource Center.

23. Answer: **D.** This term is applied across the senior living continuum to depict the aggregate customer intensity of needs (level of acuity) and scope (how many people at each level).

24. Answer: **A.** Each of the alternate response options is a subset of the correct answer.

25. Answer: **C.** An employee with reimbursable expenses must understand the mechanics of receiving payment.

26. Answer: **B.** Section 6106 of the Affordable Care Act requires electronic submission of direct care staffing information (including agency and contract staff) based on payroll.

27. Answer: **D.** There is not yet a licensing requirement in any state for the executive leader of an organization providing mainly home- and community-based services (as of August 2020).

28. Answer: **A.** The alternate response options each have more than one half of the providers in that service line sponsored by a proprietary entity.

29. Answer: **C.** The Minimum Data Set relates to skilled nursing facility; the other two alternate response options are fictional.

30. Answer: **D.** Prospective payment series for home health includes provisions for consolidated billing (except for medical equipment) and adjustments for relocations and for changes in patient condition.

31. Answer: **B.** Prospective payment series for home health includes provisions for adjustments for case mix.

32. Answer: **A.** Prospective payment series for home health includes provisions for consolidated billing, except for medical equipment.

33. Answer: **C.** The alternate response options do not pertain to the home health service line.

34. Answer: **D.** Fleet management is a form of preventive maintenance, proactively monitoring vehicular performance to foster early detection of any problems before they become expensive to repair or pose a safety threat; it is an investment in good stewardship of the assets themselves and in the protection of the lives of the people who travel in the fleet vehicles.

35. Answer: **A.** The driving performance record of each person who operates a company-controlled vehicle is the most predictive metric for underwriting risk.

36. Answer: **B.** Protecting both people and property falls under the auspices of security.

37. Answer: **C.** Elopement refers to any incident in which a person under the care of another wanders away from the grounds without the caregiver's knowledge.

38. Answer: **D.** It is possible to operate as a charitable organization without qualifying for exemption from taxation, but most providers that qualify maintain this status.

39. Answer: **D.** Each of the alternate response options describes a private care provider organization that participates in a government-sponsored reimbursement or financing program.

40. Answer: **C.** The Administration on Community Living is the parent federal agency of Administration on Aging; the National Council on Aging is a nongovernment national association; and the Older Americans Agency is a fictitious entity.

41. Answer: **B.** None of the alternate response options are agencies reporting to the Department of Health and Human Services.

42. Answer: **A.** Such permission is only granted by the CMS through approval of a waiver request, and the relevant section of the Medicaid law is 1115.

43. Answer: **C.** Punitive damages are typically awarded to a plaintiff to penalize a defendant for having demonstrated particularly egregious and wrongful conduct.

44. Answer: **B.** It is not enough to be a proficient provider of needed services in today's senior living field; conveying a genuine concern for the well-being of others must be woven into the very fabric of the organization's culture.

45. Answer: **D.** Opportunities in previously untapped locations can often be enhanced by affiliating with an entity already familiar to prospective customers there.

46. Answer: **C.** The decision to access a skilled nursing facility is more driven by need and a sense of urgency than the other service lines listed.

47. Answer: **B.** A comprehensive marketing program encompasses promotion (advertising), public relations (communicating the organization's story), and closing techniques (sales).

48. Answer: **A.** Each of the alternate response options is a quality assessment program operated by private, nongovernment organizations.

49. Answer: **B.** The National Association of Long Term Care Administrator Boards' core programs for its member licensure boards are examination development and management, continuing education approval, and academic program accreditation.

50. Answer: **D.** The National Hospice and Palliative Care Organization calls its executive leadership credentialing program the Hospice Management Development Program.

Index

Printed in the United States
by Baker & Taylor Publisher Services